Shovel It:
Nature's Health Plan

By

Eva Shaw, Ph.D

Writeriffic Publishing Group

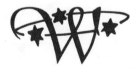

Published by:
Writeriffic Publishing Group
760-434-6445, 866-244-9047 (orders)
P. O. Box 524
Carlsbad, CA 92018-0524
www.writeriffic.com

Cover design, interior design/typesetting: Matt Shaw
Typographic specifications: Text in Times Roman, headings in Present
Photo credit: CeCe Cantón

Printed in the United States of America

Publisher's Cataloging-In-Publication
(Provided by Quality Books, Inc.)

Shaw, Eva, 1947-
    Shovel It : nature's health plan /by Eva Shaw. -
1st ed.
    p. cm.
    Includes bibliographical references and index.
    LCCN 00-111454
    ISBN 0-9705758-0-7

    1. Stress (Psychology) 2. Stress management.
    3. Gardening – Therapeutic use. I. Title

 BF575.S75S53 2001   155.9'042
                QBI00-902093

Dedication

To those who have taught me to love plants and flowers, dirt and worms, and all things that Nature shares; told stories about life and gardens; dug in the same beds with me; hauled and shoveled everything from fragrant wood chips to action-packed manure, this book is dedicated.

Laurie Blaisdell
CeCe Cantón
Vera Dooley
Ginger Hale
Ellen Hobart
CJ Johnson
Jennie Klein
Frank McKenzie
Joseph Shaw
Matt Shaw
Stella Shaw
Linda Talcott
Zippy

And hundreds of others I've met at therapy gardens, at lectures, in the home and garden center, and just out for a walk in the park.

Acknowledgments

Books don't just happen. A writer rarely wakes one morning to say, "Hey, nice day. I'll spend the next four years consumed by a topic, do scores of drafts, feel elated, feel frustrated, write until my eyes ache, write until my head feels like a ton of lead and finally have a book. Oh, yes, I'll sit for hours in front of the computer and dig through mountains of research. And when I feel it's good enough for the world, I'll throw it all out and start again." No, it doesn't happen that way.

The idea of writing a book comes about slowly, haunting the writer night and day until he or she is physically and mentally compelled to get it all down on paper. *Shovel It: Nature's Health Plan* has been that sort of book. However, without the patience, guidance, advice, counsel and great senses of humor from many, this book might have stayed a seed and never reached maturity.

Gracious and humble thanks go to my husband, Joseph, who believed in this book way back when and is now running with it, won't stop and will not rest until *Shovel It* is in the hands of every person who needs to feel better. To our son and incredible graphic designer, Matt, who produced a book and a cover well beyond my expectations. Remember, Matt, you'll never be fired, no matter what you say about my next "cute" idea. To Jacquelyn Landis, friend, colleague and the finest editor on the planet, for somehow knowing what I want to say even if my words are not doing their job.

First, last and always, for Our Father, to whom all the credit goes because only through His grace is this book reality.

Contents

Introduction

"Dig in the dirt."
"Pick a tomato."
"Smell the roses."

Do those things and you could avert a heart attack. You could reduce blood pressure and finally cut your cholesterol. You might be able to get away from antidepressants and painkillers. Surely, you'll be able to cope with the stress life throws your way.

Gardening could improve your life, maybe even save your life, says the medical community in revealing new findings published in the *Journal of the American Medical Association*. Gardening is one of the most effective longevity and health practices of our time, and that's what *Shovel It* is about.

Think of this: If you're not getting your hands dirty in the garden, you could be jeopardizing your health and happiness. You're definitely not as well as you could be. That's the truth.

Shovel It: Nature's Health Plan will make you feel better, stronger and healthier. With the *Shovel It* methods, you can tackle a score of health problems and win, while developing higher confidence, a more relaxed attitude and a positive outlook. You can improve and strengthen your heart, lungs, muscles and bones. There's ample evidence that with *Shovel It* you'll be able to toss out all those diet books and trim down to a comfortable weight. And it's free.

Read that again: It's free.

Sure, there's a catch. There are steps to achieve almost every goal, and this one includes the old accountability line: You have to do it. You, physically, have to make up your mind to implement the suggestions in this book. Yet, with the book you're holding and the recommendations inside, you can feel better, stronger and more flexible in just a few weeks. Basically, what you'll need to do is consider those things in your life that are stopping you from being healthy, happy and at peace. If you're truly willing to get well and find joy, you'll need to shovel out the rubbish that's stopping you.

With *Shovel It* you can increase your health regardless of the level you are at this very second. No kidding. No hogwash and no two ways about it.

You will have to touch the earth. You know: It's that stuff in the flower boxes, the brown-colored, gritty stuff that dogs and kids always track through the house. Seriously, that stuff that holds our planet together is the prescription for restoring your peace, health and happiness.

After you leap over that dirty hurdle, you'll find priceless rewards in your own backyard. Sure, you can do it the hard and expensive way, with programs, pills and posh health clubs. Or you can do it with a shovel and a sense of adventure.

This isn't a touchy-feely garden therapy book where you, dear reader, are able to say "poof," and suddenly from Mars or Venus or from a bowl of chicken soup, everything turns around. *Shovel It* can perhaps improve your love life, restore relationships and trim your tummy, but it's not done through a method where you whip up some hocus-pocus mantra that will make you feel like a super model or the hunk on that newest television show. No, sirree. The premise of this book is simple: There is peace, health and happiness to be found, and it's right outside waiting for you.

Medically speaking, you're about to learn how working in your own backyard, in all that soil, can offset, reduce the effects of or prevent debilitating diseases such as asthma, diabetes, chronic fatigue and osteoporosis. Are you aware that working in the garden can reduce the risk of a heart attack and restore the body after a cardiology-related episode? (That means "nearly a heart attack" in modern medical-ese.) That's what *Shovel It* promises and what you can expect.

Shovel It makes recovery after illness or surgery go faster and helps the body recover more quickly. With *Shovel It*, most people require less pain medication and heal faster. This method can help rebuild the body after a pregnancy and strengthen and restore it during and after menopause.

Speaking of emotional health, when you *Shovel It* you may discover Nature's perfect antidepressant. That's what working in the garden can do, and millions of gardeners have this as their secret to happiness and self-esteem.

There are many emotional and physical conditions that require professional assistance, so if you are troubled by issues that are too thorny, please seek the advice of your doctor. This book and the program are not meant to replace medication or essential counsel from your medical provider.

I've been gardening and playing in the garden for as long as I can remember. Wherever I've lived, I've scratched, shoveled, dug and prayed over the soil to produce vegetables and flowers. Rarely in my younger days did I give a second thought to the health-happy conditions I had created in my own life and the lives of others who shared my bountiful harvests. Then as events do, one led to another, and I could see that those who gardened were happier and healthier. As a writer who loves to do research, I began my personal quest to find out why. This book is the result of that journey, and you are about to share in the harvest, too.

Now in the middle of my life (okay, 50s, but who's counting?) and after years of studying, researching and writing about health, fitness, disabling diseases, death, grief and the negative effects of modern living, I marvel at how science has come full circle. Today, alternative therapies that are now deemed acceptable by the American Medical Association and the American Nursing Association, such as acupressure, therapy with pets, art therapy, horticultural therapy, prayer and even brisk walking, were once considered medical blasphemy.

More than four years ago, when I started to organize material for this book, I looked closely at the millions who garden. They do it for fun, to grow healthy veggies, to put flowers in their world. Gardening makes people healthy.

If getting your hands dirty doesn't offend your sensibilities, take control of your life and health. Just *Shovel It*.

More Americans enjoy working in the garden than any other pastime, and until *Shovel It*, they may not have realized how really good it is for body, mind and soul. Working in the garden is tops with scientists and doctors who quietly agree that gardening can offset everything from migraine headaches to bone loss, from road rage to recovery. After you've read the medical findings and looked at the how-tos, it's my hope that you'll give gardening therapy a chance to cure your own personal ills and evils.

What are you waiting for? *Shovel It*. You can find peace, health and happiness in your own backyard.

No occupation is so delightful
to me as is the culture of the earth.
—Thomas Jefferson, American president

Chapter 1

For Me?
Your Gifts of the Garden

There is no other door to knowledge than the door Nature opens; and there is no truth except the truths we discover in Nature. —
Luther Burbank

You're alive. You have food and shelter. You have work. You count yourself among the lucky and know those who would trade places with you in half a heartbeat.

Take a closer look. Although you lock up at night and when you're driving, it still feels safe to walk in your community. You have people around you. Some you can even turn to in a pinch or for a celebration. You have family or friends. You can vote and feel as if you have a voice. You attempt to save for retirement. Life holds comforts, even though there are some downsides to it all, and you normally feel okay about life.

Blessings counted. Let's get real.

Look at the last 12 months. They've been exhausting. Stop me if I'm wrong, but haven't at least some of the days been a struggle in one sense or another? You have co-workers, bills and traffic. How about uncooperative family members? And don't let's get started on colleagues and clients. There have been days when you feel rotten or your disposition is just plain dreadful. Go on. Fill in your preferred euphemisms. I can't do it for you, because this is a book read by all generations and it's strictly G-rated. Besides, I'm a G-rated gal.

However, I've a feeling you know me well enough already to realize I know plenty of creative terms that could apply. I've had down times and been touched with sickness and grief. As the saying goes, been there, done that.

Let's talk about you because that's what this book is about. You want to be happier, healthier and have more peace of mind. Take a chance and let's put your life under a microscope.

Does it feel as if nothing you attempted to manage (or should that be mangle?) turned out exactly as rosy as you anticipated in the past year? Forget the New Year's resolutions you intended to keep forever. They failed along about Valentine's Day—if you even got that far.

Didn't achieve buns of steel? Or a washboard stomach?

Given up gaining financial freedom by the time you saw your first gray hair?

Lost in the battle of middle management? Suddenly feel as if the clothes dryer shrank everything? Again?

Wasn't even considered for that promotion that had been all but promised?

Dated only dysfunctional types when you're seeking one to share wholesome, fun-loving fidelity with who has only a few objectionable habits?

Still can't talk to the young and the pierced that live at your house and call themselves your offspring?

Or, on a serious note, have you faced serious health problems such as out-of-control blood pressure, heart disease, weight imbalances, chemotherapy, chronic fatigue syndrome? Are you now recovering from pregnancy, glad to have your baby but tired or stressed all the time? Have hormonal surges and dips been making you crazy?

Have you recently experienced the death of a loved one, an animal companion or a life-long goal? Do you feel that your dreams are tarnished and perhaps hopeless?

These aren't your problems? Then be honest about your own jeez-it-was-a-bummer twelve months of disappointments. You have plenty of reasons to whine. Here, take time to wallow. Actually, wallowing is good for you. It's ignoring your feelings that will ultimately get you in trouble.

You're about to learn how to get rid of stress, unrest and low self-esteem, and you'll do it with a shovel and a *Shovel It* attitude.

You won't need a lot of faith to follow *Shovel It*, but you will need dirt and the determination to read through the book. *Shovel It* is gardening as therapy, and it's as easy as using Nature's Health Plan to help yourself. You must, nonetheless, take the first step. That means, spend the next ten minutes reading through this first chapter. I'm not asking for a lifetime commitment, simply a bit of your time to help you feel better for a lifetime. Really now, what do you have to lose? Could it be any easier?

> Flowers leave some of their fragrance in the
> hand that bestows them.
> —Chinese Proverb

*I think there are as many kinds of
gardening as of poetry.
—Joseph Addison*

Don't-Leave-Home Therapy

Have you been seeking an exit sign on that gridlocked freeway of life, at least during the evenings and on weekends? You'll find the directions on a packet of seeds. While not crucial to success, you can assist yourself with a trowel and perhaps a watering can, at least to start. Nature wants to guide you, comfort you through disappointments and spoil you with harmony and good health. Next time something gets you down, *Shovel It*. That's right, learn to take a new course of action and plant the seeds to your health and happiness.

Simple soil and simple Nature can help your body heal.

Here's your first of many "garden jobs." You must stop reading right now—yes, I know, you've never had a book writer tell you that before. So stop. Go out and find a leaf, twig or a flower. If you're in an office, trapped in a cubicle, quickly and quietly make your escape. If you're at home, dash out the door. You'll find a bit of nature in the garden, at the park or off the tree that's in the parking lot. Snag it and bring it back with you.

Once you get this chunk of natural stuff, touch it. Use it as a lucky charm to open the first door to the *Shovel It* method. You might want to keep it close to you as you read the next few pages. You might want to touch it and smell it and then put it aside.

This piece of the natural world will not cure your upset tummy, reduce the cost of your power bill or help you discover the true meaning of life. But if it's been months or at least too long since you and Nature have met, you need to do this garden job.

Even if you're an old hand at gardening, you must do it too. Now, don't continue reading until you've done this exercise. I'm watching, and I'll know if you cheat.

Okay, you're back. Good. And you've touched nature. Good. Now you may continue reading.

> Won't you come into the garden? I would
> like my roses to see you.
> —Richard Brinsley Sheridan, author

Think all this is just big talk from a woman who goes around with stains on the knees of her jeans and dirt on her fingers? I'm not alone in telling you that gardening is good for you.

Dr. Lauretta Young, Chief of Mental Health at Kaiser Permanente, one of the nation's largest HMOs, says, "You know, after a day in my yard, I tell my friends I have been doing 'garden therapy.' Now there are studies to prove it." The studies Dr. Young refers to involved researchers who gardened while their brainwaves were examined electronically. "What they found was that the people who were gardening had brain waves that were very similar to people who meditate." She explains that gardening actually helps your body relax. A relaxed body that's not crippled with stress will heal more quickly.

Dr. Young likes to tell of another study in which hospital patients with a garden-view room actually recovered faster. Their wounds healed about twice as fast as patients without a garden window. "And I think there's nothing more calming and soothing than the smell of flowers and the earth," she adds.

The power that makes grass grow,
fruit ripen, and guides the bird in flight
is in us all.
—Anzia Ueziersla,
Red Ribbon on a White Horse, 1950.

The premise and the prescription you'll find here in the book and in a garden is an escape hatch for the pressure cooker life we often lead.

Further, the physical act of gardening, like weeding the vegetable patch or digging holes for bulbs, provides healthy activity for muscles and mind. Garden activities such as mowing the lawn allow for stress relief and build muscles and bones. Gardening gives even the most serious-minded grown-up legitimate reasons for playing in the dirt. The garden and the physical act of gardening can be a reason, form, place and act of mediation and prayer. Gardening allows us to become connected with all that is natural and with Mother Earth. Gardening can help us restore our body to wellness.

Then there are the side effects of gardening: Organic fruits and vegetables. Herbs for natural remedies. Flowers that make you smile and decorate life. This is gardening as physical and emotional therapy at its best. All good news for gardeners. All great news for you.

It's also theorized when the brain is monitoring and controlling repetitive physical tasks (you know, the no-brainer things), it's able to connect thoughts from both the right and left sides of the brain. This makes gardening a total brain workout. Theory follows that when using both hemispheres of the brain, we have the ability to create solutions. We can work out the most knotty problems while shoveling compost. We can focus on how to have more loving relationships while trimming the hedge. We can concoct a plan for better communication with co-workers, kids or parents while weeding the petunias. We can give the brain an aerobic workout to avoid the malady that's caused by "use it or lose it." Or we can avoid thinking. Period.

In a world that's full of must-do's, not thinking for twenty minutes or three hours can feel well beyond fabulous. What's beyond fabulous? How about feeling as if you're on an all-expense-paid vacation at a four-star resort, complete with unlimited use of the room's mini bar, a uniformed driver and limo at your beck and call. And don't forget free golf, tennis, massages and room service. That's beyond fabulous.

It's as simple as answering this question: Are you willing to let Nature intercede in order to get well?

If you've answered even "Gee, I don't know," you're on the right path to making positive changes in your life. If you're not ready to make even that commitment, then answer this: What's holding you back? Are you afraid of feeling better? Please take a chance. Gardening as a therapeutic remedy for contemporary ills can only improve life.

The Shovel It method is easy.

One who plants a garden,
plants happiness.
—Chinese proverb

Show me your garden
and J shall tell you what you are.
—Alfred Austin, author and gardener

The Roots of Garden Therapy

Here are the simple "roots" for *Shovel It: Nature's Health Plan* and for using the garden to help yourself to better health.

While it works for me and many others who might attribute the whole theory to the first gardeners, Adam and Eve, I also take the horticultural approach and build on sound principles.

Gardening for recovery and improved health is much like the tiny feeder roots of plants. Want to see feeder roots? Go to the garden and dig up a plant. Annuals like petunias and pansies come up the easiest. Now gently shake off the loose soil and you'll see these minute roots. They look frail, white and tiny, but they're mighty. They're essential to the health of the plant. Now look at the other roots that support the plant. They're strong and thriving. They do their job well. With *Shovel It*, your first feedings, the first acceptance of this natural health plan, might also feel inadequate, like those tiny feeder roots. But like the roots, your connection will get stronger. It just takes a bit of time. Nature asks us to be patient.

Now back to your roots.

These roots secure a plant into the soil, bring nutrition to its stems and leaves and contribute to the production of flowers or fruit. You need roots, or a place to begin. Might sound strange right now, but don't judge. Just read.

Roots are your lifeline to a healthier future, one that is less propelled by stress and more by happiness.

These roots or steps or ideas are the foundation of garden therapy. We'll continue to talk about these steps as we move through the book: yet, they're presented here to be a lifeline to a healthier future.

- ❀ Accept Nature as an all-knowing force. Nature will supply the ability for you to start those feeder roots, if you give her a chance, because there is a time for every purpose under heaven.

- ❀ Open yourself to Nature and Nature's lessons. Look at the seasons as a road map for the cycles of life and the cycles of your own being.

- ❀ Ask Nature for help with your garden and your life. Ask out loud. So that your family and friends don't think you've jumped off the deep end (wherever that is), you may want to talk to Nature while you're alone in the car or shut in the bathroom.

- ❀ Give thanks. A simple, "Thanks, Nature," will do. She provides the trees, the flowers, the air, your life. This is true even if your world is imperfect right now.

- ❀ Look to the underlying forces in Nature that are all around you. Begin to notice how Nature affects your life from wearing a hat on a windy day to choosing the most succulent produce at the market.

- ❀ Share your ideas with other gardeners as they, too, open up to Nature and open their lives to you.

- ❀ Allow yourself to feel at one with all of Nature's creatures: birds, mammals, the tiniest of seedpods to the largest redwoods. Do it for one minute. Yes, you can check your watch to make sure you're not over-staying your welcome. This exercise will help you begin to find a place for Nature in your heart and mind.

❀ Work in your garden as a gift to Nature. She will give back to you many times over.

❀ Refuse to give room in your garden for private fears and hidden demons (those voices that say "You have a black thumb" or perhaps, "You've always been a failure"). Never allow them to halt you from learning and enjoying all that Nature provides.

❀ Get out of your own way. Stop trying to make everything just so. Nature teaches us to have real expectations. Bad things do happen to good people. Sometimes plants and people die. Even people we love and who love us get angry, hurt and feel vengeful. Some leave our lives.

Flowering plants wither. Frosts and floods hit vegetables. We fail and have disappointments. We do and say thoughtless, stupid things, and stupid things are done to us. But there's always next season—always another try and another time.

Make it a practice to use all your senses to communicate with Nature.

> *Nature is just enough; but men and women must comprehend and accept her suggestions.*
> —Antoinette Brown Blackwell, *The Sexes Throughout Nature* (1875)

It seems that everything in life comes with directions. Even the directions on a can of Campbell's soup tell cooks to open the can. *Shovel It: Nature's Health Plan* has directions, too; however, these are much like the rules for making a sandwich. They have to do with your own taste.

If you were making a hero sandwich, you might put some of this stuff on it, and you'd never forget to add that stuff. I like green olives, cucumber and avocado. Another sandwich maker might say, "Get that green stuff off—this is a real sandwich," and then load on the pepperoni, hot salami and jalapeño cheese.

Tastes in sandwiches and gardening are varied and personal. Nonetheless, since most of us work best when we have an objective or can see the goal post, even if that goal is vague, here are the directions:

1. Forget all the rules you've heard about gardening.

2. Do what feels right for you.

3. Challenge yourself. You're the only one who counts.

4. Follow the directions that you want to follow. Dismiss those you don't, but expect the garden to change you.

All my life through, the new sights of Nature
made me rejoice like a child.
—Madame Marie Curie

Anyone who has a bulb has spring.
Bulbs don't need much light; they don't need
good soil, and they don't need cosseting.
They are, in fact, the horticultural equivalent
of cats: self-contained, easy-care and
supremely suited to living in New York.
—Anonymous

What to Expect

Expect the best when you invite Nature to work in you and through you in the garden. She wants you to have

Peace

Love

Health

Harmony

Along with sex and food, these are the things most of us strive to attain. Begin now to think of gardening objectives and desires. How do you "see" your garden? Does it come anywhere near that of which you dream? Why? Why not?

As you work through the book, you can expect to better understand the connection between you and the universe. You might even begin referring to Nature as God, or vice versa. If talking about God and your garden is uncomfortable, you might consider God an acrostic, which stands for Good Orderly Direction. Because that's just what you'll get when you ask for help.

Expect to wonder about your future and the future of your garden.

Expect to know with your heart oftentimes more clearly than with your brain.

Expect to cope with the unexpected. No matter how impeccable you are with the dahlias, trust me, they'll get some type of bugs or disease. Marauding neighborhood dogs (maybe your own) will visit your lawn and produce spots on that lush green carpet. Without even a second thought, the wind will rip off the autumn leaves just before they turn that screaming scarlet you've been waiting for.

Of course, you can stomp your foot and shake your fist, but you'll end up like most gardeners. You will shrug and think, "Next year." That's one lesson of the garden; it teaches us to know the future as more than possibility.

To be with Nature puts you at risk of becoming optimistic. With each attempt, taking chances becomes easier. This is part of the healing process. In taking chances, whether it's with a plant or your health, you look to the future and have the faith to plant again, love again, restore your health again. Nature teaches you to be a risk taker.

Expect to believe in miracles.

Small miracles do happen in your garden once you have the eyes to see them.

Early yesterday morning, outside my kitchen window I noticed a rose cane shooting toward the sky. It was one of those basal canes that rose lovers covet. It was fat, thick and vibrant. With the first cup of coffee, I casually noted the cane was about six inches from the top of the fence. By noontime, it was nearly to the top of the fence. This morning it's inches beyond the top. Even though I sneaked into the kitchen, never once did I see it grow. Did it only sprout when I wasn't watching? I call that a miracle, but perhaps I'm more open for miracles than some people. Perhaps you will be, too.

Big miracles take longer. If you're using the garden for weight control or stress reduction, you may get a hint of the feel-better future in the first days. But the rewards will take a bit longer. They need to be cultivated and cared for just like the peas, corn, pansies and calla lilies. If you're using the garden to lower blood pressure, manage cholesterol, reduce the need for pain medication or build strength after chemotherapy, cardiac arrest, a debilitating disease or serious physical condition, your own growth and return to health may feel slow, but it's happening.

Like that rose cane, you may not be able to see the changes as they happen, but over a period of time they will be dramatic.

Expect to have to look for miracles. They won't all be as apparent as the first crocus popping through the snow or the first blue jay snapping berries off a bush.

While working in the garden, my feelings switch between sheer bliss (we're talking that exploding wonder-of-wonders stuff) to sweaty mindless suffering. Sometimes when troubles happen, I force myself to get out there and get my hands dirty. It's not always fun, spiritual or recreational. It's not always because I want to. Some garden chores are daunting and hard work.

Some days I rationalize that it's not worth the bother and it's too messy. Why garden just a few minutes and get yet another pair of sneakers muddy?

It's these times that I must push myself out the door. I go without a plan. I don't think, "Oh, this is so healthy for me. I'm strengthening muscles. I'm promoting higher levels of HDL (the good cholesterol) by increasing activity. I'm going to sleep better tonight. La-di-da!" That's a bunch of compost.

When I'm in a funk, I don't care about brainwaves and rejuvenating cells. I don't care about weight control or strong bones. I don't think about these things, but I force my feet to get out to the garden.

It's then that I sit in the garden, and flawed as it is, I look around. If I think, which I don't often do at these times, my mind might go on to philosophical questions regarding the connection of Nature and my emotional balance (or imbalance), my place in the world, life in general, my presence in the cosmic soup of life and so on.

I could theorize about the imperfectness of my garden as a metaphor of my life. I don't. When I'm suffering with a case of the moody blues (whether it's physical or familial), I don't rationalize well. Do you?

Life and gardens are alike, of course. Yet, Zen and the art of gardening doesn't come to mind when I am waging a war with myself, someone, something.

Maybe you have experienced this: There are times when I mentally "duke it out" as I sit in the garden, on the grass or as I hack away at a bush that threatens to take over the walkway. These are the times when life makes no sense at all. Have you ever noticed that as we get older and supposedly have the answers, the questions get thornier?

It's times like these when I grab a stick or a weed to shred into a zillion pieces. I may get down and fanatically yank at the Bermuda grass, which constantly invades my garden.

Speaking of weeding, it's a perfect form of therapy if you're looking for something truly mindless. I've discovered when weeding that I can find a flicker of relief whether I'm suffering from terminal writer's block or physical maladies. Psychologists might call it pouring out frustrations. No, sorry, weeding doesn't help solve all of life's problems. If that were true there wouldn't be a weed anywhere in my garden, and this book would be called Weed Therapy. However, gardening, especially weeding or any repetitive physical activity, can get you out of yourself, just for a second.

That's the first twinkle of acceptance in the process the brain uses to cope with a change. The change could be physical or emotional, such as the death of a loved one, and that act of acceptance slowly transforms the disaster into one we can acknowledge.

There are times when I'm sad and disillusioned. Then I find myself drawn to walk around my little suburban plot. I do laps. I look much like a prisoner strolling the compound.

Then a shift happens, not every time, but often enough as I walk through the garden. I move from "poor me" to "I didn't see that shoot on the apple tree." I stop punishing myself or others for some real or imagined and more-horrible-than-possible fault, just another of life's dreadful misfortunes, and look at the colors in Nature.

My mother, Jennie, could stick a twig in the ground and it would grow. I remember her saying, "Just look how Nature planned that all her flowers would never clash."

What does that nugget of maternal advice mean? Could it be simply that you can put an egg-yolk yellow Marguerite daisy next to a wine red Mister Lincoln rose bud and shock the senses, but the rose and the daisy never collide?

Or perhaps she was telling me that opposites, even impossibilities, can coexist if we're smart enough to see and believe in the connection. The coexistence can become stronger if we're aware of what's happening.

If I'm especially introspective, I realize that I can coexist with the problem or person consuming my thoughts. I don't have to agree, like it or even understand it, but I can live with the condition or the difference.

Expect the garden to surprise you, challenge you and disappoint you. The garden is your life. The garden is about life and living.

> You have to pick the places
> you don't walk away from.
> —Joan Didion,
> A Book of Common Prayer.

Listen, God loves everything you love
—and a mess of stuff you don't. But more
than anything else, God loves admiration...I
think it pisses God off if you walk by the
color purple in a field somewhere and don't
notice it.
—Alice Walker, The Color Purple.

Call Me Ishmael
Or Whatever Name You Choose

Can Nature (The Power, Universal Energy, God or any other name you're comfortable with) solve all our problems? Right now?

How I wish that were true. Can Nature help deal with pain and loss? Is it really necessary to examine how Nature works? Must we look any further than acknowledging that it feels right when we let this goodness into our hearts and work that therapy through our hands? To most of us, life is a mystery and there's mystery in life. Perhaps it is just so in Nature.

Nature wants us to be happy. Nature wants us to understand the cycles of life. Nature can get us through even the most challenging times if we merely look, listen and smell what she provides. Nature gives us reminders of that power in a monarch butterfly, the first daffodil dressed as if going to a *Gone with the Wind* ball, and the crisp crunch of autumn.

When those times come where there's more chaos than answers, it seems natural to turn to other people or turn inward and away from Nature. The garden can't solve credit-card debt. It's crazy to think that Nature can return a loved one to health or soften the searing pain of grief. It sure as shootin' can't fix a broken heart. Or so we think.

Hey, come on. We're grown-ups, we can cope. We can get angry. We fight back. We can figure it out on our own. Now get out of my way.

Yet Nature continues quietly along, presenting solutions with simplistic lessons. Nature reminds us every day of a world that stretches beyond a disappointing job, a terminal illness, an ill-fated romance or the death of a loved one.

While the wonders of Nature and gardening as therapy have been known to us garden-variety types for eons, it's only been recently that medical science has said, Hey, maybe there's something there.

In an article published in the *Journal of the American Medical Association* (November 11, 1998), a survey found nearly half of all Americans would choose to be involved in alternative therapies (such as gardening) to ease depression, anxiety and chronic conditions.

Further, in another study documented in the journal, medical researchers in Sweden tracked groups of patients, all with similar reasons for hospitalization. One group of patients was assigned a room with a painting of a garden. A second group had paintings of forests in their rooms. The third group had geometric abstract artwork on the walls. And the fourth group had no paintings. The first group—the ones who looked at paintings of gardens—recovered faster, needed less pain medication and reported less depression than any other group. Those with the forest scene did second best. The group viewing the abstract art needed the most painkillers.

Let's walk into your garden in order to consider this. Let's focus on the power of Nature and draw some conclusions. If just looking at a painting of a garden can help hospitalized patients feel better and have less pain, and if looking at a painting of a garden can help our loved ones, friends, family and ourselves get well more quickly and suffer from less depression, what might time spent in a real garden do? I've thought about this for a number of years in the garden, while leading bereavement groups and facilitating recovery sessions, and when talking to friends.

Please ponder this for a moment.

Gardeners know the answers. Now you know, too.

Some gardeners, like those who merely cut the lawn on Saturday and trim the shrubs in the fall, may not have considered these implications. Others keep the whole thing a huge secret and smile a lot.

Now, if this information doesn't get you back to your roots, at least to the point where you begin to wonder, then you need to read the results of the study again. Go on. Nature is always patient.

> There is material enough in a single flower
> for the ornament of a score of cathedrals.
> —John Ruskin, author

Gardens, like people, are living, breathing entities, with personalities that are distinctive.

Some look as if they're scowling back at us, just like some people do. Some gardens are bleak, nearly barren of life, or so it seems on the surface. Then a gardener comes along to nurture, plant, water and care for that once dismal place. A miracle? It took nourishment, attention and time. Isn't that what we all crave? Have you wanted a pat on the back but didn't get it, a good word but got a grimace, a hug but received a frown? Yes, we've all been there, but Nature never responds in those ways.

Rather, a barren garden tells of potential, the flourishing one talks of contentment. Nature shares the messages, and when we're listening, shows us how to hear and see. Nature's Health Plan guides us to feeling better.

Gardens are connections to a world greater than our own, and in turn we can restore ourselves within the confines of a garden. They give us hope. The garden teaches us faith (or to learn to believe again) in ourselves, our world, our planet. The garden underscores the lessons of life from how to share and listen to ways of being gentle, patient and introspective.

The garden and Nature show us how to start over, how to manage, how to forgive and how to take chances. The garden is the ultimate therapist and offers the supreme recovery program. If we can create our dream garden and live in it, at least in our mind's eye or heart, we can begin to create our dreams of life and live them, too.

We can understand, just as Nature reminds us every day and throughout each season, that a garden is never complete. It is never perfect, nor are we. Native American lore dictates that in every basket, bowl, rug or hut, there must be a mistake in the workmanship. To do otherwise would be blasphemy to the Great Spirit.

A garden continues to prove this lesson. There's always work to be done. Whether we think so or not, Nature wants us to learn by success and failure.

> Hope is the feeling you have
> that the feeling you have isn't permanent.
> —Jean Kerr, Finishing Touches

Some time back, Walt moved into my neighborhood. His home is along my daily walking route, and as gardeners always talk to new neighbors, we struck up a friendship. Walt does stuff with computers, a software developer or engineer or guru or something.

I didn't see him for a while and assumed he'd lost interest in the garden, until one day strange things began to happen, at least strange for his neighborhood.

Lawn, which had once stretched in a glossy emerald mass, was ripped up. There were mounds of topsoil and a California oak—a baby one—appeared. I still didn't see Walt. Since I walk by at the crack of dawn, I didn't really expect to see him working there, but curiosity was getting the best of me.

A week later herbs appeared: yarrow, feverfew, verbena, thyme, rosemary. I'm sure a few neighbors were horrified by the sudden disappearance of the front lawn. But then a vibrant herb garden took its place. I loved it all.

After what seemed like months, I did meet up with Walt. He was happily puttering among the herbs, checking out the new lily pond. "I need to know," I said. "Why did you put such a non-traditional garden in such a typical suburb?"

The story unfolded. In the months I'd not seen him, Walt had suffered from Bell's palsy, facial paralysis and extremely high blood pressure. A tall, trim man in his forties, you'd think he was an athlete, not someone with chronic health problems.

"Blood pressure that was so high, my doctor was concerned about a stroke," Walt said handing me a chunk of rosemary to crush and sniff.

After months of trying to reduce his blood pressure with drugs, aerobic exercise and yoga, all to no avail, Walt stumbled on gardening as a way to relax. "My doctor is still amazed but won't say for sure what made the difference. But I have proof that gardening lowered my blood pressure. I'm supposed to monitor my blood pressure every day, and I've documented the results. I found that nothing—the medicine and the complicated workout—helped like being in the garden. When I'm working in my herb garden, surrounded by the plants, fragrances, the sunlight and the soil, my blood pressure becomes manageable. The positive and stress-reducing effects last, too, even when I have to deal with problems at work and in life."

Walt wasn't a gardener before the garden called him to action. He doesn't know the plant names or all the rules. And he knows some of the plants will thrive while others will die, and he shovels those straight to the compost heap. There are no rules for gardening, and no beginnings or end. Could gardening and Nature have saved Walt's life? I think so, but then I'm a gardener and know the benefits of *Shovel It*.

At this time in your life, and the life of your garden, just stop. Really, stop all activity. Spend five minutes or ten trying to clear your mind. Often we're so busy (dishes, reports, runny noses, e-mail, you name it) that we forget just to become dormant. Plants remember, trees remember, the grass turns brown.

Right now, turn brown.

If you're living or working with demanding people, schedule a time in the next twelve hours to be alone. Do not wait longer than twelve hours. You deserve to feel the yearnings of dormancy (regardless of the month of the year). It's time to release tension, forget about should've's and need-to's.

Become alone in your self and trust that you will find a new comfort level. It's okay to go into the bathroom and lock the door if that's the only way you can have a private moment.

Sit in one place. Do not move. Try not to think. Just be. Nothing is expected of you.

Stay. • Be. • Exist. • Breathe.

Right now you are experiencing a cycle of life and of the garden. Be still. You are waiting. You are resting. This is Nature's message as we move through the seasons, repeated yearly, to our subconscious, to our hearts.

Focus your eyes to see stillness. Ecclesiastics 3:1-8 gives us Nature's lesson:

To everything there is a season and a time
to every purpose under the heaven: a time to
be born and a time to die; a time to plant,
and a time to pluck up that which is planted;
a time to kill and a time to heal; a time to
destroy and a time to build; a time to weep
and a time to laugh.

Imagine the connection with the earth, clear and strong. Rest and open your arms, pull in Nature's essence. Move away from thinking and struggling and calculating. Move inside your internal garden, that beautiful place in your heart where you are totally safe. What do you feel? Why do you feel this way?

Those who dwell, as scientists or laymen,
among the beauties and mysteries of the
earth are never alone or weary of
life…Those who contemplate the beauty of
the earth find reserves of strength that will
endure as long as life lasts.
—Rachel Carson, naturalist

A Garden Growth Exercise

As soon as you can, go outdoors. It's way past time to feel a stronger connection with Nature, so sit down right on the earth. Actually, now is the perfect time, but you can wait until this evening, or if you must, wait until this weekend. Don't skip this gardening exercise. It's essential for your growth and helps you put down your roots so you can experience Nature's goodness.

You can go to the park, the lake or seashore or in your own backyard. Put your face down near the grass, sand or dirt. See the world from a bug's viewpoint.

Now turn your head and look at how immense other creatures are. Your dog or cat is mammoth. Did you see the size of that seagull? Pebbles and blades of grass are massive. A fence is gigantic. The trees are colossal. You are tiny. You are insignificant. You are negligible.

Now slowly unfold and stand. See and feel the world shrink. You are master of this environment. You are not the minuscule scrap of insignificant being hovering for safety close to the earth.

Spread your arms. The world is your garden. You are powerful.

What are you sensing? Responsibility? Self pity? Painful memories? Physical suffering? Do you feel connected to your self or cut off from feelings? As we connect with Nature and our self, we become larger inside. Our heart's garden grows. Yes, it needs to be nurtured, but even now we can feel accomplished, we feel a kinship to all that is in Nature.

Nature wants us to thrive, to have our health restored and to feel in charge of the world, as you did when you stood up from the ground. Nature provides a way to bring beauty into our lives and into the lives of others.

You have just accomplished the first therapeutic exercise. Part one was when you felt your being shrink. You were a bug's size. You could have easily been crushed beneath a human's foot, blown astray by the wind or drowned in the rain or the sprinkler's burst of water.

Some of us go through our lives feeling insignificant, inadequate, small and incompetent. Some of us feel as vulnerable as a bug.

What a waste. Why feel insignificant when the feeling can be changed?

You just saw that by changing perspective (standing up), you needn't be a victim of your surroundings, your life, your world. You are strong. You have roots. You can change. You can grow and bend and be more than others think. You can be more than you think you can.

Change your perspective and change your life.

*A cheerful giver doesn't count the cost of
what he gives. His heart is set on pleasing
and cheering him to whom the gift is given.*
—Julian of Norwich,
Revelations of Divine Love, 1373.

Say What?
Why Are You Too Busy to Hear?

Do you have dreams? Do you nourish them? A garden is a parable for dreams, and if you don't believe this, talk with gardeners. They see what the garden will be long before reality sets in.

I fantasize that my garden looks like something out of a Thomas Kincade painting. Note the word fantasize because it would take a crew of gardeners and boat loads of money (neither of which are mine in reality) to make that dream happen. Yet, as other gardeners will tell you, we enjoy shoveling it. We dig in the soil amendments and know we'll never really get rid of weeds, yet that doesn't stop us. We keep working.

A dream in development is a vague plan that gets called to action once you visit the garden center. It starts when you pull out your wallet, take out a charge card or write your check for the things you must have. Most gardeners dream of perfection but experience real life with bugs, slugs and other assorted garden problems and pests. Nonetheless, dreams continue.

To dream, you must have time to think and be alone. Are you spending enough time with yourself? Many are not if they are in the middle of a tension-filled time, such as during an illness, juggling parenthood with person-hood, coping with a trying relationship or staying in an uncomfortable career.

We may also attempt to organize every second, perhaps unconsciously believing that if we stop, the true answers will turn from whispers, heard just out of ear shot, to shouts we won't be able to silence. Some watch too much television, party too much, drink too much, dash from one sexual encounter to another. Why? It's easier, or so it seems.

Those whispers and shouts, the "voices" that I believe are Nature's way of telling us we need to find inner peace and improved health, are one of my favorite topics when talking about gardening, garden therapy, health and recovery. Recently, after speaking to a large group on this very subject, a woman waited patiently to speak to me. After presentations many people want to share a bit of wisdom or a story; some want to ask personal questions. This woman stood to the side and waited. When her turn came, she took off her glasses and delicately took my hand. "I'm a psychiatrist, honey. If you hear voices you had best get some help."

Sometimes I'm concentrating so much on the new friends and gardeners I'm meeting that it takes a moment for words that don't fit a situation to sink in. Then the meaning behind her words finally connected into my brain. Sorry, but I know I chuckled, then, thanked her and silently vowed to continue to listen to my voices. She wasn't a gardener, apparently, and just didn't get it. I hope you will.

We all realize that there are people who have serious problems and need to get medical help. If you or a loved one is among this group, assistance is available. That's not what I'm talking about here when I'm talking about listening to your voices and your dreams. Please don't misconstrue the meaning.

I'm suggesting we should all listen to the garden-variety voices that start in our hearts. I believe that Nature, or God if you prefer, is communicating with us in this way. It's an intuitive language that's comfortable, if somewhat quirky.

Nature is gentle and won't lash out to give advice. Rather, her whispers are in the breeze, in a squirmy worm digging through inky loam, and in a rainfall on a splattering sunny day. To be healthy and grounded, we need to listen.

Sure, we could hear it in our own voice and with our own word choices. And we could hear it with the voice of famous folks. But let me tell you, I'd freak out if suddenly the voice of Humphrey Bogart, Bette Davis or John Wayne began talking to me about Nature's Health Plan. I'd lose no time finding the doctor who tried to counsel me after that workshop.

Nature might be quirky, but I think we're safe from hearing Bogie in our heads.

Try this now. Sit for a few minutes and listen to the voices in your head. Ask yourself these questions:

Am I so involved in work that my plants, loved ones, pets and friends are shortchanged? Be honest, because they may not have whined.

What have I been neglecting, in the small picture (taking out the trash) or in the big picture (doing the creative work that's secretly in my heart)?

Do I feel my healthiest? Am I comfortable with my body?

Are there habits (or things I do) that need to be addressed so I can feel and look my best?

Do I feel that I look too old for my age?

Where are my dreams? Why have I forgotten them? How should I nourish those dreams? Do I know how to get started? Why haven't I started?

Who do I allow to usurp my energies? Who are these people? Why do I allow them to do it?

Do I give up my energy, time, money, personal space because I've always done it that way or because others expect me to do so?

If you've followed any of these patterns for a while, you'll probably hear (or have heard) those voices in your head. Are they saying mean things? Unprintable things? Calling you a wimp or worse? This is Nature's way of getting your attention—you are not crazy or losing it. This is her Health Plan.

Just listen. Just learn. Give Nature a chance to speak to you by shutting off your outside responsibilities and those which take away your power. As you begin a physical, spiritual and emotional gardening program, you may need to transform or stop some behaviors. You'll let them go in order to make room for the new, healthful ones.

Be aware, starting right now, that when the feelings or the negative behaviors surface, you'll need to tell yourself, "Stop it." Say it like you mean it, too. Slam a palm to the table, look yourself squarely in the mirror. Get serious. We believe what we hear out loud. Shout it out. Try it now: Stop it.

> Desperate ills need desperate remedies.
> —Agatha Christie,
> The Mystery of the Blue Train

Take on one task in your garden, or your life, and do it as well as you can.

It might be as simple as mowing the lawn every Saturday, using the blower to clean the snow off the sidewalk or organizing the tool shed. Maybe your task is to cut a few flowers or a sprig of pine for the desk, mantel or table.

Could you rake a few leaves? Snap off some faded blooms?

Even if your task is to walk around a public garden or the park, you'll experience a feeling of accomplishment.

As you do this work, give yourself credit for overcoming small hurdles that have stopped you from being a part of Nature. Too often in our high-tech world, we are so apart from the soil in the garden that it seems almost deadly. Sure, there are exceptions and toxic dumps, but most of the time, the soil that's in the garden (or around trees and planters in the park) could be far cleaner than the money you touched when you bought a donut or a bagel this morning. So it's okay to touch the soil and let it trickle through your fingers. Try another handful if the first feels good. You might feel more relaxed just by this simple connection with Nature. Many do.

When you begin to change and listen to Nature, another transformation may have to take place. You may need to become involved with others who didn't know you before. Getting involved doesn't mean you have to devote your life to "good work." It can be as simple as taking a class, joining a group or simply listening and being with others who know your gentleness.

You may want to become a friend to the aging trees in the city park, volunteer with the Audubon Society, design a garden next to the emergency room at the local hospital.

You are not alone. Millions suffer, many silently, from physical and mental and emotional traumas. Millions falsely believe that their problem or situation is unique or so terrible that if anyone out there knew about it, they'd be ridiculed.

In Nature's world, nothing is terrible. If you give Nature a chance, she'll be there. Yet, if your feelings, body or well being are unmanageable in any way, there is help. Talk to a listening friend, consult with your clergy, make an appointment and see a therapist. You're probably suffering needlessly. You may need a chat or some sunshine. Do not feel you must face fears or the unknown alone.

Nature's lesson is clear: Stop. Look. Listen. Be. Ask.

Still, in a way, nobody sees a flower, really,
it is so small, we haven't time, and to see
takes times, like to have a friend takes time.
– Georgia O'Keeffe, artist

Bug Juice

We share this planet. Use organic methods of pest control whenever you can. Here's my recipe for "bug juice" that's toxic only to pests. In one gallon of water, mix 2 tablespoons baking soda, 1 tablespoon white vinegar, 1 tablespoon dish soap, 1 tablespoon light cooking oil. Pour into your garden sprayer and spray for aphids or powdery mildew—do not spray during the heat of the day or in direct sunlight. Morning sprayings, well before the day gets warm, are the best.

Because this recipe for bug killer is non-toxic, it's safe for those undergoing chemotherapy and those who may be sensitive to commercial sprays or concerned about the environment. I especially like this because it's safe to use around pets and children, although I make sure they're not close by when spraying.

When I was most tired, particularly after a
hot safari in the dry, dusty plains, I always
found relaxation and refreshment in my
garden. It was my shop window of
loveliness, and Nature changed it regularly
that I might feast my hungry eyes upon it.
—Osa Johnson, author and adventurer

You Need 'Em.
Do These Garden Jobs

❁ Get some gardening magazines and seed catalogs. There are gardening magazines and catalogs online and at the store. Ask gardening friends for their recommendations.

❁ Using magazine photos that are expendable, cut out your favorite plants and flowers from the pages and paste them onto a poster board. Look at how the colors combine. Analyze the textures of the plants. Will a cactus really feel okay next to foxglove?

❁ Read one book on gardening. Check the library, the bookstore, your own shelves or an Internet bookstore for selections. Ask gardening friends for their favorites. Even if you've never had luck growing African violets, that doesn't mean you can't learn about them, and in that process find out how to nurture them. At the back of this book is a suggested reading list of my favorite gardening books. Start your own list, your own library.

❀ Go to the nursery or one of those huge garden centers and buy an inexpensive houseplant (under $5). Yes, you can buy online, but it won't be quite the same for this exercise. You'll have plenty of time for online shopping, you really will. You might be tempted to pick one up at the grocery store when you stop for coffee and tissues, but don't do it. The nursery or garden center is a field trip for your well being. Be selective, but allow your heart to rule your decision as to which plant to choose. This isn't a head decision. If there's an incredible gloxinia that's beckoning you or a maidenhair fern that's yanking your heartstrings, plunk down your money.

❀ When you've picked your plant, talk to it. Talk to it on the way home. Talk to it when selecting its location. Sure others might think you've gone off the deep end, but do you really care? I hope not. Give your plant a pet name, like Boris, Spot, Jack or Pinkie. Call it Morning Starlet, Butch or Celestial Phoenix.

❀ Read about your plant so that you know how best to care for it. Make a note in your daybook or on the calendar or in your journal as to when you purchased the plant. We'll talk more about garden journals and photo journals later, but if you're ready to take on one of these projects, flip to the index for some suggestions.

❀ Sit down next to your plant and look closely at the vegetation and the flowers (if it has them). Notice the delicate coloration. Have you ever seen so many shades of green? Feel it working to bravely cope with a new environment. Sense its resolve to survive and thrive. Help it to do so.

❀ Know that same resolve is in you.

The best place to seek God is in the garden.
You can dig for Him there.
—George Bernard Shaw

Chapter 2

Get Your Hands Dirty

Everybody needs beauty as well as bread,
places to play in and pray in, where Nature
may heal and cheer and give strength to
body and soul alike.
—John Muir, naturalist

Nature doesn't keep a scorecard, and there are no rules for her therapy. Since that's true, you might be seeing it as one big, natural free-for-all of green stuff.

Sure, you could dive in willy-nilly and plant anything or everything. Lots of gardeners do it that way.

The trick, however, in creating a garden that has therapeutic value is to select plants and flowers that reflect you and your gardening dreams and feelings.

All therapy gardens should have places for you to:

sit

pray

dream

think

unwind

rewind

nourish

your spirit and your soul and your body.

It's everything that slows us down and forces patience, everything that sets us back into the slow cycles of nature. Garden is an instrument of grace.
—May Sarton, author

Let the Journey Begin

Want to have a connection with Nature? That's what she wants, too. She also expects you to be dependent on her for guidelines and to learn. No rules, mind you, but recommendations. Think of Nature as your mentor. Or maybe the best friend you've always wanted. She's a great listener, always supportive and nonjudgmental, too.

If you live in one of the temperate zones, or you and Nature have already become pals, consider yourself fortunate. Your approach to a therapeutic garden may still take time and may even require you to rethink your ideas and your gardening goals. Just like you can't lose forty pounds by next Tuesday at four o'clock, regardless of what Internet sites and television commercials imply, Nature's Health Plan takes time and thought and energy and tenacity and love. Did I mention that you'll increase your patience in the process?

Let's say you live in Tucson, Arizona, with mild winters but summers that can be compared to fire-engine-red, blistering chili salsa with extra dashes of Tabasco straight from Louisiana. But you've been dreaming and coveting and fondling the idea of a garden filled with ferns, delicate columbine and spikes of blue delphinium.

Perhaps you live in a city's high-rise or a condo without a scrap of green. You're thinking of a luxuriant garden room that's filled with earthy smells of moisture. It's that same fragrance you've experienced walking into greenhouses at the nursery or public garden. You're dreaming of a place to replenish your soul.

Or you live in Buffalo, New York, and have simply gotten adjusted to tons of winter that covers your backyard, your sidewalk, the bus stop and your life from November to mid-April. Yet, you find hope and comfort in images of lushly exotic vegetation in your perfect therapy spot. For you there could be nothing so soothing as orchids, plumeria, bougainvillea and succulents, along with the cologne of red ginger wafting through your senses.

Impossible dreams? Silly objectives? Out of the question? Not at all. Even if you live in a climate zone that is unsuitable for a certain plant, odds are you can grow it where you live. So first off, let's get this straight: There are ways you can achieve your consummate therapy garden regardless of the climate or your lack of garden space. The catch is that you'll need to collaborate with Nature and stop fighting her efforts.

You're going to have to spend more time creating an environment that's special, but your therapy garden will be worth it.

When mentally pondering your garden, focus on the following. Be truthful because you can't fool Nature. What is:

❀ your time commitment?
❀ your location?
❀ your budget?
❀ your yard, balcony or windowsill's size?

❀ your need for a garden?

❀ your specific challenge? (Voracious deer, energetic kids, neighbors who are too close, rocky soil, bricked-in patio or garden apartment, lack of air quality, noise pollution.)

With a garden that's designed for many purposes, from an active play area for the kids and the dogs to an outdoor extension of your home for entertaining or writing or painting, you have choices. You can design a portion for yourself for therapy. It might be a meditation corner. It could be a wooden bench beneath a fir or maple. It might be a niche near a fishpond or a birdbath or your swimming pool.

Work with plants, flowers and art in unexpected elements to comfort and soothe you, to awaken and influence you. Whether you're working with an established garden or starting out fresh, the choices are not even limited by those six items. But you're going to be limited if you think of failures, inexperience or supposed inadequacies. Willing and praying and pleading with dead plants to regenerate won't do any good. The same goes for self-defeating thoughts.

To make a garden a place to de-stress and get healthier, you must shovel out dead, inappropriate or unappealing plants. This could be a parable to life. When we're ready to get healthier and find increased self-worth, often we must change situations, jobs and even relationships. You have, or will have, a relationship with your garden. Shovel out what's hurting it or you, and put in the things that make for a healthy life.

What you shovel out or what you leave in is your decision alone. Of course, there may be specific dictates: a swing set for the kids, a grove of fruit trees, a humongous tree. We all have constraints in life; some can be managed, some must be moved aside or put in order to create new life and new beginnings.

Keep in mind that everything is fair in gardening.

Nonetheless, with gardening therapy as your objective and a shovel in hand, you can transform even the bleakest spot into a place for therapy and happiness.

So right now, instead of working out nooks and crannies for the garden where you can find tranquility and happiness, health and joy, where you can sit and make heads and tails of life, stop and consider the process. The journey to discovering your garden, designing a gardening and maintaining your garden, is a gift to yourself.

Sure, you could, if you have the cash, write a check to a garden architect or landscape specialist. Lots of folks do it, but that's not the point of gardening as therapy.

If you hire someone, you'll have to be a good communicator of ideas and feelings. You'll have to explain the therapy garden concept and what plants, flowers and features you like. It's up to the expert to make a plan. Let's stay with this fantasy of "money's no object." The end results, if all is right, will be that you'll have a garden that is tranquil and inviting.

Still, you'd be missing the point, the pleasure and the therapy of shoveling and using Nature's Health Plan. The physical acts of creating and sharing Nature's job cannot be hired out. You must do it yourself.

I don't think of my garden as a place only to produce flowers, fruits and vegetables. Yes, I love to share the bounty, and I've yet had anyone turn down a bouquet of Double Delight roses or a bundle of oregano. But the entire concept of selecting, transplanting, nurturing and learning to take chances is part of shoveling out the chaos of contemporary living and inviting peace and health into life.

Working with Nature, I've accepted the risks and the consequences, coped with failure, and flaunted and savored in positive results. You, too, will feel part of the process if you give it a chance. If something is not doing well in the garden, many will wait one more season to see if it responds, but after that, it's shoveled.

Your garden will never be perfect. Life isn't. Nevertheless, the process of gardening can satisfy you more deeply than writing a check to that landscape expert.

Even if you believe you psychically zap plants and flowers with a horticultural death curse, I urge you to try again. Nature is a forgiving, loving mentor. She'll take you back no matter how often you kill plants. Really.

If you are absolutely not lured to connect with Nature at the most basic of levels (like getting down on your hands and knees planting seeds), or because of a disability you cannot do it, then get help.

If you hate the idea of Nature's Health Plan, I'll expect a letter from you saying that you've just proved me wrong, and you cannot enjoy the gardening process. The therapeutic and healthful value of getting your hands dirty didn't work, and you're still as troubled, tired and angry as ever. Now that you know you can contact me and grumble, gripe and moan, or you can complain to Nature of the unfairness of the world, I urge you to give this drug-free therapy a try.

*Since I am convinced / That Reality is in
no way Real / How am I to admit / that
dreams are dreams?
—Saigyo Hoshi, Japanese Poet*

There has been no creation. How can there
be "the beginning"? The creation is
continuous; it is creativity. Back you move,
you will not find the beginning, ahead you
go, you will not find the end. It is
beginningless, endless creative energy.
—Osho, author, Discourses.

Welcome to Fantasy Land, Your Garden Meditation

Nature's Health Plan has begun. It's time to plant the garden of your mind and heart. For this exercise, you'll need a comfortable, quiet spot and a pencil and paper. You'll need your imagination.

Read over the meditation process that follows, and then close your eyes and visualize your garden. After you've felt the garden begin to come alive in your mind, jot down some notes about it or draw a sketch of it.

Be aware: This is the ultimate garden that you and Nature can conceive. While it can become real, at this point it need not be based in anything even close to reality. I'm not implying that you rush out and attempt to duplicate this meditation and make it the genuine article, unless that's physically and financially possible.

Your goal right now is to feel the presence of the garden in your heart and mind. Even if you've never experienced gardening, trust the meditation to create a garden in your mind. This is a no-holds barred exercise. Actually, you may want to do the exercise a few times, in various moods, to find a garden that feels right and accomplishes many purposes in your life.

The plan needs to filter through your conscious level. Let your flight of fancy go wild. That is, you may "see" a lily pond with koi, hear the tinkling of a waterfall, smell a conifer grove richly decorated with fragrant blue spruce or view an elegant English walled garden where trumpet flowers cascade over the mossy stones. You can have your garden circled by a picket fence with yellow and white Simplicity roses clustered just to the sides of the waist-high gate. There might be arbors, swimming pools, outdoor fireplaces, a magical play area for the kids or an elaborate patio for outdoor dining. Don't dwell right now about what others will think. Yes, be selfish. Think of you.

Relax and take some slow breaths of air. Expand your abdomen and your lungs. Try to clean out all the worries and responsibilities of your life—at least for the next five minutes.

Read the narrative that follows. Then close your eyes and dream.

When you're ready, scribble your garden ideas on that paper. Some people make lists and take notes. Others use colored marking pens and draw pictures.

> The trouble with gardening is
> that it does not remain an avocation.
> It becomes an obsession.
> —Phyllis McGinley, author

When I have trouble writing, I step outside
my studio into the garden and pull weeds
until my mind clears—I find weeding to be
the best therapy there is for writer's block.
—Irving Stone, author

The Meditation

Feel the breeze on your face. It's not too warm or too cool. The air is soft and creamy, like peachy-smooth, vanilla-laced whipped cream.

You can now walk into the garden, and you see it like an artist's blank canvas. The potential is everywhere and you feel powerful. Should you sit on the bench that's so tempting, or plunk on the grass or nestle in the spot where the earth is exposed? It's up to you.

As you make yourself comfortable, whether it's in the shade or the sun, a garden will appear. You feel it before you actually begin to plant the plants, the flowers, the trees, the extras that make it your own dream garden.

Inhale. Exhale. Drink in the potential that abounds around you. Need a hint of what you'll be smelling? Think of the fragrances you smelled the last time you walked into a nursery or a glass arboretum or a public garden. That's what I'm talking about here.

What do you see? Planters? Flower beds? Tubs of tulips? What colors are predominant? Lavender? Scarlet? Hot pink? Icy blue? And the texture and variety of plants and the flowers. What mixes did you conjure up? Are there grass, rocks, pathways, a stream and an arched trellis with a gate? What stands out most? What did you see first?

Now begin.

Once you have a clear picture of your mental garden, or the garden in your heart, if you'd like to use my terminology, you can revisit anytime you need to relieve stress or feel more connected to Nature. Even if you can't physically go to or sit in the garden, this garden of your heart can be visited anytime you need it.

The very next time you're upset, unwell or troubled, go to your heart garden, breathe in the fragrances, and you will feel more relaxed. Sound too easy? Why not try it?

> Weather means more when you have a
> garden. There's nothing like listening to a
> shower and thinking how it is soaking in and
> around your lettuce and green beans.
> —Marcelene Cox,
> Ladies' Home Journal, 1944

You may want to make some notes about this pie-in-the-sky garden. You might want to revisit it and make some changes. You might want to sketch it out. Flip through magazines to find some ideas on garden plans close to that which you've seen in your meditation time. Many paste these images or photos on poster board or make dream garden collages. This, too, can be a way to feel connected with Nature, especially if winter is making everything ungrowable.

Is your fantasy garden anything like what you honestly have now? What aspects can you snatch from this meditation and include in your real garden? Take five minutes and jot down your ideas or make some sketches. There's no wrong way to do this exercise. You are in the discovery stage.

When I did this exercise, my secret garden was sunny, bright, and overflowing with flowers. I am addicted to flowers of every kind, and in the meditation I realized that all the flowers in that garden were pick-able. Since I have the joy of living in San Diego, gardening is a year-round blessing. As I write this, Thanksgiving is tomorrow, and looking out into my garden I see roses, bird of paradise, daisies, snap dragons and morning glories still in bloom.

Flowers are my passion and my undoing. That's my gardening criterion and what I discovered with the meditation. There's nothing I love more than picking bouquets. I love to have bouquets in the house, to take to church, to share with friends and to give away in unexpected ways, like to the woman who owns the cleaners, or to my dentist and my hairdresser. I like to make theme-color bouquets, such as those that include a secret message in the flower-speak that we'll talk about shortly. I like to create mixed bouquets with the unexpected, like peppermint or peppermint geranium added as greenery.

I like to design therapy bouquets with flowers that traditionally heal, mixing feverfew with roses, adding a sprig of rosemary. The recipient may not know that for centuries herbalists have been making remedies from these flowers and plants, may not even know why smelling and seeing the bouquets makes one feel better, but they do. That's good.

I believe that Nature works with me to create an engaging flower garden, and I work with her to share that splendor.

Now get your nose into the action. How did your fantasy garden smell? Okay, I know it was designed in your mind, but take the plan a step further and concentrate on the fragrances you'd experience if you were actually in that garden. Did it smell moist and fertile like the floor of the forest or the earthy scent of mushrooms? Was it sweet and drenched in essence of honeysuckle? Did you smell the fresh, clean aroma of sunlight on piney greens? Could you smell the tomatoes or the aroma of berries?

I love fragrance in the garden, and when visualizing my fantasy garden with this exercise, I realized that the perfume of flowers needed to be included. While I might lust after a pretty bloom at the nursery, if it can't promise to please my nose, it doesn't come home. Why not? I won't be satisfied and I'll *Shovel It*. Time lost, money lost, and precious garden space lost, too, says the voice of my experience.

Now let's check the colors. What colors did you see? Green? If so, you've just discovered a valuable clue. Nature is suggesting lots of landscape plants, perhaps a low-maintenance garden with plump bunches of herbs, vegetables or grasses and hearty scrubs. This garden is restful to the senses, a little on the wild, unkempt side and drenched in mellowness.

If there were flowers galore, jot down the shades and the names, if you know them, but don't fret if you can't tell a crocus from cyclamen, clarkia from a canna. (There are plenty of reference books and websites that give access to horticultural dictionaries and experts at the garden shop to help you out with the particulars.)

As we'll talk about later in the book, color is an important part of the garden. Don't neglect this aspect. Briefly, for a peaceful spot, you'll want to select flowers, vegetables and herbs in the range of blue, white and purple. For an uplifting, busy and happy area, you'll want to select flowers in the red, orange, pink and yellow range.

Now let's look at where you'll hang out in the garden. What about the furniture in your fantasy garden? Where did you sit? What did it feel like? Were there wooden benches, wrought iron tables and chairs, cushioned nooks, a worn and inviting tree stump?

With whom did you share your fantasy garden? And did you see and feel wildlife there? Did you envision birds and bunnies? What would you like to have cohabitate with you in your space? Bees? Butterflies? A toad abode? Food for squawky jays? A shelter for squirrels?

All the things you have visualized will in some way mold the style of garden you begin to select or transform.

In my ultimate fantasy garden, there's greenery everywhere. It's a walled kitchen garden with sheltered paths and inviting vegetables, which seems at odds with my love of color and flowers and gardening projects in progress. I like space in my fantasy garden with a bit of lawn. There are benches, a brick walkway and a birdbath large enough for the crows to bathe. There's sunlight and shade. And best yet, I don't have to see a neighbor or share it. Sometimes sharing is overrated.

Now back to reality. My suburban plot doesn't match this vision, not by a long shot. Most likely yours will not either. That's okay. Don't allow the disparity to upset your plans. The fantasy garden is the beginning of your reality garden. With luck, plans and your shovel, you will be able to transform parts of your fantasy into the world in which you live. With Nature's help and your imagination, you can see gardening dreams come true.

What did you learn from your meditation? Are you more comfortable with the idea of creating a garden? Did you discover that you want huge rocks or tiny plantings, overflowing buckets of herbs or a spa surrounded by a redwood deck smack dab in the middle of it all? With your notes and your sketches, with your fantasy and your reality, you've begun to make your impression a reality. Enjoy the process. In times of unrest, or when you can't sleep or if the pain is becoming too much, go straight to your dream garden. It'll help because now the journey is underway.

*Is the fancy too far brought, that this love
for gardens is a reminiscence haunting the
race of that remote time when but two
persons existed—a gardener named Adam,
and a gardener's wife called Eve?
—Alexander Smith, author*

What's Your GP?
Discovering Your Garden Personality

No two gardeners use the garden in the same way. It's more than the potayto-versus-potahto argument, it's reality. And we're about to get very personal, so if you blush easily, keep in mind that the answers to the following will be confidential.

You may want to take the assessment twice: once for your personal, inner desires and another time to connect with what you must produce to share with your family members, those folks who routinely think of you as mom or dad, grandparent or relative.

The results of the assessment can help you focus on what you want in a garden, and specifically on what healthful or de-stressing uses you plan for it. There are no right or wrong answers. But your answers may get you to think about your needs for a garden where you can feel free and relax, unfettered by the demands of your job, family or the world. It should be a place where just you and Nature can be on first-name terms, even if it seems like you're arguing sometimes.

Go through the following questions and write the appropriate number next to the answer that is most like you.

Write:

4 if it's most like you or what you want with your garden.

3 if it's somewhat like you or somewhat like you want.

2 if it's occasionally like you or occasionally like you want.

1 if it's not at all like you or never what you want in a garden.

A. I enjoy being outdoors.

B. You'll hear no cursing if my hands get dirty or my knees and sneakers
   get muddy while I'm in the garden.

C. I always manage to have time for the things I enjoy, including relaxation.

D. I like that feeling of satisfaction after exercise or time outdoors and in the sunshine
   or fresh air, without regard to most of the weather Nature sends my way.

E. I like to play outdoor sports or did when I was younger.

F. Money is a consideration, but I seem to manage to budget for those things I want.

G. Some people have said I'm persistent.

H. I rarely think of myself as hard to please.

J. I can laugh at myself.

K. Life has thrown some failure my way and yet I've bounced back.

L. There's something restless going on inside me, and it seems time to add
   a new hobby or way of thought to my life.

M. Recently, I've had a significant change in my life, such as the loss of a loved one, an animal companion or a job. Or I'm retired, about to graduate, or considering some life-changing prospects.

N. I'm trying to contend with a thorny, formidable situation at home, work, school or in my life.

O. As a child, I liked to climb trees, watch the clouds for patterns, swing from a jungle gym and daydream about far-off places.

P. I often find color and texture exciting. I've been known to crush herbs to drink in the flavors or gather leaves in the fall.

Q. If I had to make a choice, I'd choose reds and pink over green.

R. I've never considered myself a neat-nick, where everything has to be in its place.

S. If I have time, I enjoy walking or participating in an exercise program.

T. I like to read and often relax with a book.

U. I have friends or family who garden or know about gardening, organic produce and fresh herbs or flowers.

V. When traveling, I have visited public gardens, art museums, or wildlife areas. Even on a hectic business trip, I've been known to walk through a park or do laps outside of the convention center or hotel just to get some fresh air.

W. I would like everything in apple-pie order, but a bit of clutter or chaos is okay.

X. I know that tomorrow is another day.

Y. I take time to admire Nature's wondrous work.

Z. I'm concerned about the environment and worry about what earth will be like for future generations.

Scoring:

There are no right answers to this gardening assessment; however, the following may help you form a clearer picture of your garden and how you see gardening as therapy.

85 – and higher: Active GP. You're an energetic individual with an impatience that's well blended with the acceptance of imperfection in your life. You may be in the midst of a traumatic situation or recovering from an addiction or loss of a love.

You see the garden as a hobby that's fun, burns calories, and gives you a sense of creating beauty. Most likely you strive to add color, texture and sunshine in your yard. Be sure to arrange for a sanctuary. This can be as easy as a shady spot where you'll pull up a chair and be alone or where you might spread a mat and do yoga. It can be filled with tropical plants or exotic vegetation. It might be a fragrance area where you can use the plants and flowers in aromatherapy treatments to help you restore your mind and body. If you're an apartment or city dweller, this sanctuary could be a tiny rock garden where you will always keep fresh flowers or flowering plants. Or perhaps you can stake a claim to one of the plots in your city's public garden. Begin planning your garden, a place for therapy and fun.

65 - 84: Spontaneous GP. Sometimes you enjoy being active and see yourself as having a good sense of humor. You can joke about your shortcomings and even after a major hurdle can find a hint of humor in the situation. You've been known to say or think, "Someday, this'll make a great story," and then add a shrug.

You've weathered a trauma or two and would enjoy having a garden that's tranquil, perhaps a place to retreat to when the world begins to close in.

You're not afraid of getting dirt under your nails, and the idea of working in the garden, along with those repetitive tasks, such as weeding and shoveling out a new garden area, holds interest for you. You know at least one gardener or bona fide garden nut. You may dream about how you can improve your own garden, the pots on your windowsill or the public garden you've visited.

A garden is like life. Life is always changing, and so are the plants, flowers, vegetables and trees that you're sharing with Nature. The garden is never perfect, yet will nudge you to believe that someday you can achieve near perfection. Gardening tasks are never over.

When planning your garden, with the tips and ideas found in the Garden Bubble, you will want to share your space. Don't make it so prissy that kids, dogs and your clumsy cousin Chip, in-laws or a neighbor can't enjoy it, too. You'll probably want to include a birdbath or bird feeder, perhaps a patio fire ring, or install a putting green. (Did I just tempt you? Great.)

> 45 - 64: Tranquil GP. There are times when you want to lie back and block out the world, but know you'd be missing too much love, joy and friendship, and besides, denial never really works for very long. Look to the repetitive and nurturing tasks in the garden for help with your problems and quandaries in life.

Because your "perfect" garden is one in which you can relax, put your feet up and enjoy the flowers, vegetables, herbs and other plants, make sure you tuck rest areas into your plan. However, design the garden for your health and happiness as well as to share. You'll want a singular space for you and more room to entertain and to create parties. You may want a meditation or prayer area. Be sure to include ideas for cushioned patio furniture, even if you have to bring it in at night.

The secret way to locate the right spot for meditation and prayer, and perhaps a few yoga stretches, is to take a blanket or cushion, sit there for a moment and then move it around to another location in your garden. I can't tell you how you'll feel when you find the place, but you'll know it. If you're concerned with noise pollution, such as the highway too close or the airport within screaming distance, consider installing a waterfall or dense hedge. This could reduce the noise level that turns you away from the garden.

As you work on the Garden Bubble when planning your garden, remember you're not the only one who will be using it and admiring it. Make it fun. If you're too serious about the garden, you'll probably become frustrated and thus lose the benefits of finding health, peace and happiness.

You're not the type of gardener to be a slave to delicate plants and flowers. Make your garden easy to maintain.

    Under 44: Individualistic GP. You're somewhat reserved, focused, idealistic, and well, okay, I'll say it: You're picky. Has anyone said these things about you? You know in your heart that if the world were the way you would have created it, everything would be just so. And you also know that it will never be that way, and that's part of your frustration.

In the past, gardening has infuriated you since there were no guarantees that what you planted would live, that you would like the result of all the hard work, that what you paid for would even work. When thinking of your garden, you'll want to select ultra-low maintenance and nearly foolproof shrubs and trees. You'll want to design and install a drip watering system on a timer so you don't have to be concerned with one more responsibility. If you're not the handy type, have a contractor do it for you.

When designing or improving your garden, add pots of colorful annuals mixed with herbs such as chives, rosemary and basil. Again, select the low-maintenance ones, or buy the pre-made pots of herbs or annuals straight from the nursery. As you brainstorm and get creative about the garden and therapy you want, make good use of the natural elements already in your yard.

Check the index for recommendations on shady gardens and those that get lots of sun. Design your garden so you can see colorful flowers or plants when you pull into the driveway after work or through a window over morning coffee. This will help your feelings of peace and revitalize your patience.

No act of kindness,
no matter how small, is ever wasted.
—Aesop, The Lion and the Mouse

Get It Off Your Chest

Step 1: Don't skip this section.

Step 2: On a piece of paper (or in a journal) write down a minimum of ten of your likes and at least ten of your dislikes (petty and otherwise) about gardening. Get it off your chest. Love the flowers? Hate the mud? Love the trees? Hate to rake leaves? Love homegrown lettuce and carrots? Hate the gooey slugs? If something about gardening really frosts your cookies, pour it out.

I love it when God has plans for my garden and brings the birds, who carry the seeds that grow strong and tall in the garden that I tend. For instance, sunflower, lantana, violas and even trees have come to me in this way. I recently discovered a crop of tiny Italian Stone Pines smack dab in my rose garden, which I transplanted to a more appropriate spot. That's one joy of gardening—discovering the unexpected. But it's not all a bed of posies.

I hate putting insecticides and pesticides in the garden, hate to assassinate snails with the latest and greatest killer on the nursery shelf and have been known to hate people that pour the stuff on like it was somehow good for us all. Now don't get me too riled, but you get the picture—and it's not pretty.

These are poisons, and I believe we share this planet. While I know there's a place for pesticides in responsible gardening and agricultural programs, I try to do without. So—and you may have guessed the punch line—my flowers, bushes and trees have blemishes. Pesky green worms have munched the roses. Until I found a natural deterrent, the daffodils were fair game to slugs. One year, the Liquid Amber had, horror of contagious horrors, white fly. I could practically feel them spreading to the Bird of Paradise, the Silver Maple and the Loquat tree. Life went on. Even if I added a few more gardening wrinkles to my furrowed brow.

I've had to lower my standards and figure out how much cohabitation I can handle with the pests of the world. And I've had to learn non-toxic ways to keep my garden as pretty as possible.

On this list, write what you hate and write what you love.

Step 3: As you work physically in your garden or as you plan it, refer to this list. For instance, if you can't tolerate the concept that bugs have walked on the lettuce you're adding to a salad, don't grow lettuce. You don't have to grow vegetables. If you can't stoop over to tend a flowerbed, plant in tall containers or in baskets.

Nature's lesson is that all gardening is therapy. You're in charge of your own future. Your ideas, wants and desires count. This is the way it's supposed to be. Nature is here and wants to nurture you, if you'll give her a chance.

For instance, in my garden, I have a fragrance bed with herbs, mint geranium, rose geranium, mint, violets, lemon verbena and fragrant annuals, all in the same area as an old-fashioned and incredibly prolific climbing rose, Cecile Brunner. I go for good smells here. There's a portion of the garden dedicated specifically to the roses to which I'm addicted. It's in the middle of the backyard and edged with brick. In the front of the house, I have a raised bed that I like to pretend is an English country garden. Okay, the truth is out. If you come to visit you'll have to use imagination, just like I do, because this garden is the size of four postage stamps but chock full of annuals and bulbs that are staggered for blooming from January through December. I change the color theme and display with each season. I put in ceramic garden elves and add annuals. I have been known to *Shovel It* all and create a nearly instant rose garden. I'm practical when I'm wearing the career hat of a writer, mentor, speaker and teacher, and I'm capricious as all get out in the garden. Heck, I'll do whatever my current fancy dictates, based on the balance of my gardening budget.

In the areas that are transitions from the front garden to the back, there's low-maintenance Wandering Jew, with tiny sapphire flowers throughout the summer. Until last year, on the west side of the house where there's cozy afternoon sun, I allowed the nasturtiums, lantana and geraniums to take over where they thrive in the less fertile adobe dirt. Recently I shoveled it, put in barrels of soil amendments and there's now a rose garden. (Yes, more roses.) I walked through this area not too long ago and noticed that the nasturtiums are coming back, a welcome sight for any gardener's eyes.

My garden isn't a show place. *Fine Gardening* has never called begging to do a photo shoot. The words well-groomed and Eva's Garden are not synonymous. When you visit you'll see a pile of firewood stacked for winter, a picnic table, a garden bench, fruit trees and room to play ball with my dog or have a picnic on the lawn. We love to eat outdoors. Nearly every lunchtime we pull out beach chairs and picnic with our soup and sandwiches. We move the chairs around the garden, often bringing along the Sunday papers or a cup of strong coffee or bottles of homemade root beer. Notice this isn't a sissified garden. It's tidy and nice and supremely usable. It's functional and goes with my ever-changing desires. It is a gardener's garden that always needs work, is ever changing and always holds potential.

Others have different ideas of their therapy garden. Meet my friend Gloria. Gloria's garden is immaculate and down-right spectacular. She frets over the slightest color change in foliage. If a prized plant looks peaked, I imagine her calling 911. She frets, worries and gets into a full-blown snit if a visitor hints that she may be too addicted to gardening. Yet, she receives immense joy nurturing, talking to and coaxing her charges. She daydreams over her garden, too, seeing in the plants the shapes and designs of her experiences. Gloria's garden is on a windowsill at the convalescent home where she's lived for the last eight years. She grows air plants, tiny kalanchoe pinnatas and bryophyllum that cling to scraps of driftwood her children have brought from the rocky coastline in front of the beach home where she once lived. Until the car accident that left her paralyzed and that produced seizures so severe that she's unable to care for herself, she gardened in the unforgiving, sandy soil of California's northern coastline.

Now those memories are erased, but the urge to experience Nature remains strong. "In the window sill garden, in these institutional surroundings, in this place for those less fortunate than me, I can garden. That makes me happy." This is what Gloria tells visitors who come and say they are family, but whose faces she doesn't remember.

I'm often asked if Nature can work miracles in the garden. For years, my instinctive answer has been yes. Then I found proof. When some four dozen patients who had recovered from cancers that should have been fatal were surveyed for the book *Remarkable Recovery*, it was found that most of these patients believed that their prayers, meditation, faith and exercise had produced their recovery. They believed and produced a fighting spirit, reported the physicians.

This theory is directly applicable to your recovery in your garden. If you have faith, if you meditate and pray, and if you actively exercise while in the garden, perhaps even the scourge of illness can be defeated.

Create your garden. Make it your own.
There are no rules.
—Anonymous

The Garden Bubble

Welcome to the reality portion of *Shovel It: Nature's Health Plan*. Your counselor, Nature, wants you to form a plan that can help you succeed. She wants you to create a place where you can get exercise, fresh air, and find tranquillity. She wants you to form your goals and add beauty, good vegetables for the table and the body, and exquisite shrubs and trees for the world. And she'll help you do it.

You already have ideas about your strong points as a gardener, which you got from the Gardening Personality assessment. You may even have thoughts on what really should constitute your ultimate gardening experience, possibly inspired by the garden meditation. By now, you're pretty clear on your likes and what you want to avoid in the garden, and with a little more information you'll be ready to design or make some changes in your backyard.

Get this straight: Unless you have unlimited money or a wealthy relative who dotes on your every desire (and will supply unlimited funding to your projects), you are not going to be able do everything you want with your garden at once. Some of the work you'll encounter includes the following:

❀ Manage the process of gardening. We're talking schedules, seasons and budgets.

❀ Understand that in gardening, as in life, compromise is necessary, even when we don't want to.

❀ Focus on the big picture as you're digging rocks the size of the planet Mars, trying to rid the backyard of a cactus garden, or managing the spring (summer, fall or winter) storms that make you feel as if you're living in a swamp. You'll have to have patience.

At work or in school, you may have used various methods to brainstorm and come up with creative ideas or to discover new products. Sometimes this is called clustering or mind mapping. I call it "bubbling."

The trick with bubbling as a method of brainstorming new and creative ideas and solutions is to avoid censuring yourself and the innovative ideas that zoom in from no known hemisphere of your brain. Nothing you can come up with is stupid. Nothing is impractical. Nothing should be thrown out, at least initially. This is the way creative discoveries occur. I now understand that Leonardo da Vinci is said to have used it. I thought I'd invented it. Regardless, bubbling is a potent garden tool.

When I'm mentoring tentative or new gardeners (those who can't tell a petunia from a pansy) I love to share this technique. Master gardeners find it beneficial, too, because many of these pros get muddied down in tradition, and bubbling lets them free their creative souls. This plan is so simple that everyone catches on quickly.

The object is to look at your yard (or windowsill or community plot, which you hope will become your garden, too) in a fresh way. Your first "go through" should be the pie-in-the-sky dreams, maybe ideas collected from photos in magazines, maybe visions generated from your garden meditation. From this first draft, you'll select those items that are somewhat reasonable for your second draft. On your third draft, you'll again select the best of your plan.

If you're unsure about the types of gardens or specific healthy natural touches you want to add, flip further ahead in this section and read about garden types. It's okay, really, because in the garden nothing need be permanent, and it's okay to be fickle. You can have a little of this and a lot of that, or vice versa. Your garden can be a buffet of floral and vegetable and shrub and tree delights—or whatever delights you at this moment.

What are the lessons Nature is trying to teach us? To be flexible. To cope with blemishes. To discover comfort in the proximity of perfection. To say Again. To say Yes.

Those new to gardening should know,
however, that most gardeners hate to part
with dirt, clay pots, pickle jars, really good
labels, stakes, tarred twine, and any kind of
wooden box. They do not mind giving a
plant that sells for $40 if they have an extra
one, but the other stuff
(which may be worth a dime) it tears the
heart to part with.
—Henry Mitchell, gardener,
columnist, author

All the buddhas, bodhisattvas,
and enlightened beings are present
at all moments to help us,
and it is through the presence of the masters
that all of their blessings are focused directly
at us…All we need to do to receive direct
help is to ask.
—Sogyal Ripoche,
The Tibetan Book of Living and Dying.

Now let's bubble.

Here's all you need to know and do:

1. Buy or find some large pieces of paper. You can use a child's drawing pad or the classified section of the newspaper if you want (although when I do that I get distracted by the ads). You need big sheets for the best result.

2. Get some colored marking pens or the crayons from your children's art box. You'll want to use many colors, perhaps even illustrating ideas as you go through the process. You are not being judged for your art ability. You are not being judged at all.

3. Draw a circle in the middle of your paper.

4. In the circle, print the words "My Garden." (If you want to illustrate inside this circle, do it. Ivy would look good. Yellow daises around the edges? Well done.)

5. Draw ten lines radiating out from the circle. It will resemble a child's line drawing of the sun.

6. Draw a bubble at the end of each of these lines.

7. Print ten features inside the end bubbles that you think you may want to include in your garden. A feature might be a vegetable garden, a Bible theme garden, a meadow, a planter with herbs, a greenhouse for orchids, a sundial, a bird feeder, a flagstone patio, a rose-covered arch, a group of brightly painted rocks or colorful bottles, shells strung in a wind chime effect, a homemade maypole or a flock of pink plastic flamingos.

8. Don't censor your ideas. This is an exercise where the wilder your ideas become, the better. It's brainstorming. You're not to go near a nursery or shovel or landscape computer program yet. You'll have time. As a matter of fact, you'll do better if you do this exercise before you take any of the "reality" steps.

9. If ten circles are not enough, do more. You don't need to show this to anyone —it's potential, it's creativity and it's all yours.

10. Now, with a new piece of paper, place each feature you've identified in a center circle, and repeat the process. For instance, if garden art is in one of the circles, print that word in the middle of a clean piece of paper and begin to brainstorm the types of garden art you visualize being included in your garden. You might see spiritual statuary. You might want to envision cheery painted signs. What about something totally whimsical like oversized military boots, purchased from a thrift store, filled with cascading lobelia or violets?

11. Now hang your garden bubbles on the wall. Place them where you can see them. If you've ever pondered which wallpaper to put in a room or what color to paint, you know that it helps if you paste a slip of paper or color chip up and live with it for a few days. That's what you need to do with the bubbles. Some of the ideas you brainstormed might seem odd or even weirdly wonderful. Some might seem ridiculous or totally outrageous. Some might become downright dull, yet you won't get the feel for them unless you complete these steps.

You might find that the silly turns into perfection. So what if you find that you're dreaming of a totem pole in the middle of what you'd planned to be a kitchen garden.

If you're thinking of planting vegetables, such as squash, tomatoes and beans, you'll have the basis for a Native American garden theme. These were the big three sources of food for America's first peoples, our Native American tribes. That totem pole will feel right at home.

Having no rules for your garden bubble is a crucial part of your therapy. You are creating. You are pondering. You're working on mental images and seeing if they can come close to your reality. Please don't rush this process. Some people take a few days to weeks to live with their ideas and watch them transform into a workable plan.

Take whatever time you need. Nature will wait—she has all the time in the world. Realize you may hear a whisper or two while she's waiting, but that's just the way Nature operates. Besides, Nature wants you to be happy. If you're not, you will not succeed.

It's time to wonder and meditate on your own body, your physical self, as a feature in your garden. Do you see yourself in the process, working the soil, tending that which is in your care? If you're not in this mind's-eye picture, why not? What's holding you back? If you cannot visualize yourself in the garden and surrounded by Nature, fresh air and all that grows, take a few minutes to return to the Garden Meditation. Place yourself in the middle of your dreams. Then return to the garden bubble.

Now with your heart and mind's eye look at your garden from all angles, even from your windows.

Japanese philosopher and poet Hsueh-Tou saw and spoke of life through the window. "What life can compare to this? / Sitting quietly by the window, / I watch the leaves fall and the flowers bloom, / As the seasons come and go."

What do you see through your window on the world?

12. Take your bubbles down off the wall, putting these plans away for a day or a week or two weeks. Think of the plans, but don't look. It's too soon. After a week or so, return to your bubbles and study your ideas.

Some may be shocking. Some may be too timid. You may want to make changes.

Ask yourself, "If it weren't impossible, I'd…" Why are your choices impossible? Cost? You'll find lots of inexpensive ideas in this book and other books. Space in the garden? Think small. Think containers. Think about getting a space at your community's public garden.

Do you fear creative ideas? Creative urges? Ideas that seem to fly in from another dimension? Sometimes it's scary, but it's always true: We honor Nature and the Creator when we are creative. Nature wants us to create an enchanting garden or garden spot. She wants us to have a place to relax, get physical, nurture and feel at home. Can you truly deny Nature the pleasure of seeing you smile, dream, rest, unwind, lounge, contemplate, plan, and combine what is around you to develop a more beautiful world?

13. Selecting those features from your bubbles that feel right to you, make a final bubble. This may be your long-term and ultimate plan. Be patient. Nature doesn't expect you to build and create it all in one day or even one year. Nature is steadfast, and she believes in you. That belief is unflagging. She is forgiving, loving, giving and helpful. Give her a chance to help your garden grow.

14. From this final Bubble, make notes, design it further using one of the garden landscape computer programs, or draw your ideas on a tablet. You don't have to be Van Gogh. Just do some rough sketches. Hold off. You need not share these ideas with anyone. You're in the creation process, and some people will not understand.

See your ideas come alive. Keep the Bubble available and look at it often.

15. Expect to create and you will. Expect this garden therapy work to soothe your mind and it will. Expect Nature to produce new ideas seemingly out of nowhere, sometimes during dream times at night. Expect to succeed, and succeed you will.

In the next chapter, you'll find ideas and practical help for garden features and designs, but first you have another garden job. This requires time.

*Sweet flowers are slow
and weeds make haste.
—William Shakespeare*

Time
An Essential Garden Job

Time.

Time to dream from your window.

Time for action.

Your job now is to discover and create ways to make your Garden Bubbles come alive. Your goal is to make the ideas jump off the paper.

At this point in the creation of the garden, it's time to daydream. Flip through landscaping books, garden design books, books and magazines at the bookstore or library. Feast in the photos and find joy in the prose. Check out the options available at online garden supply sources.

View the ideas as a challenge and source of natural joy. Then turn your ideas over to your practical self. That is, if you like wrought iron sculptures, in your mind and as conceptualized in the ideas produced from your Garden Bubble, see what these pieces of art look like in reality. Some may take searching, but you can find examples. This is part of your recovery using Nature's Health Plan as therapy.

If you haven't yet bought or started a garden journal, get one now and begin to write in it. You'll need to keep track of your ideas and thoughts.

Take a field trip and visit a large garden center or outdoor landscape center that sells art, rocks, furniture or gardening displays as well as flowers, vegetables, shrubs, exotics like orchids and trees. See the types of garden materials. Take a pad and pen to jot down the types of features and items each store has, and check out the prices.

Check out software on garden design. Attend home and garden shows. Watch the gardening networks. Subscribe to the free online gardening newsletters. Subscribe to magazines and begin a garden scrapbook. Read about the parts of gardening that are a mystery or the parts that you adore. Gather ideas.

Take matters into your own hands and scribble your feelings of the features along with ideas on how you can individualize your garden in your journal.

Flowers and plants are silent presences;
they nourish every sense except the ear.
—Mary Sarton, author

Chapter 3

The Garden
of Earthly Delights

We are co-creators with God,
not puppets on a string waiting for
something to happen.
—Leo Booth, Creation Spirituality

Have you ever stopped at a flower stall to ogle the blooms?

In a lightning bolt of nearly childlike enthusiasm, have you felt the power as you put your entire face into a bouquet? Think of the fragrances. No perfume, regardless of the price tag, can duplicate those scents. Are you aware that with little or no previous gardening training at all you can create, with a little time, that same perfume in your backyard?

When was the last time you plucked a piece of fruit from a tree or snatched a strawberry from its shelter of green leaves? How about digging radishes or carrots straight from the earth and scrubbing them off beneath the garden hose? Can you taste the juice, the freshness so succulent that words can't come close to describing that essence? Yes, you can grow fruit and vegetables, even on a balcony in the city.

Now think about those wild meadows or savored memories of childhood that were part of teenage daydreams. I remember them—cascading reds and oranges, huge clusters of Queen Anne's Lace and sunny yarrow. Meadows just made for fantasies of daring maidens and handsome knights on white horses.

When I was a youngster, my Uncle John and I hiked the mountains that embrace Santa Barbara, California. It seemed it was perpetual springtime. At least that's what comes to mind in my memories, and though decades have passed, the vibrant, creamy purple lupine dotted with hot orangey California poppies, acres of them, still radiate in this reminiscence. It's as if those days have been engraved on my heart and can be recalled and loved time and again, and I've long thought about recreating the vision in my garden. Do you have such memories?

Finding meadows in our towns and cities may be a thing of the past, but we can replicate them in our gardens by creating wild areas, filled with blossoms and naturalized grasses.

Now it's time for more of the gardening tools that will help you shovel out some things that are not healthy or no longer reflect the healthier you. Allow your garden's image to become sharper, as if you're focusing binoculars or wiping mist off your glasses. As you do, consider how your garden can and should be a place to reflect on life, as well as a place to play at living. Let the fun fill you. You needn't have a reason, but you do need to know what Nature expects.

In this chapter you'll discover must-know stuff about the gardens in your life, such as thrifty, creative ways to get more plants for your garden and make new friends. We'll talk about keeping a gardening journal and about specific gardens designed with your therapy in mind. We'll talk formal gardens, trendy/arty/whimsical gardens, tropical and Oriental gardens, mobile gardens, those wild meadows, scent gardens, hanging gardens and a whole lot more. Within each brief garden description you'll also find tips on how to make the most of the therapeutic effect of gardening.

For instance, if you've ever dreamed of living in a jungle paradise, the tropical garden would bring much more potent therapy than working in a low-water, low-maintenance desert one. If you're allured by the idea of Zen and the Art of Gardening, then an Oriental garden is a must have.

No need to make up your mind yet. Read the descriptions. Ponder the verbal pictures. Do the planning exercises. If possible, take a field trip to a garden center, decorative stone yard or quarry to see the enchanted pieces of rock that Nature has available for your garden.

> My good hoe as it bites the ground revenges
> my wrongs, and I have less lust to bite my
> enemies. In smoothing the rough hillocks, I
> smoothe my temper.
> —Ralph Waldo Emerson

The green metal chair is an indispensable
piece of equipment. As Farmer Bagley
said, "How can you grow anything without
a chair? How else can you see
what's going on?"
—William Longgood, gardener and author

Your Garden Journal

For decades journaling has been recommended by psychologists, social workers, the clergy and other helping professionals as a way to understand thoughts and figure out issues that trouble hearts, minds and bodies. Today, women and men are writing in journals without the urging of the medical community to record creative thoughts, keep lists and notes and record dreams, hopes, joys and nightmares. Writers keep journals, as do poets, parents and other prose-filled individuals.

Gardeners have long used notebooks as a place to record just what's going on in the garden and to document changes, the flowers and plants and trees and vegetables that work, and those that need to be shoveled. It might be something like this:

May, The Clematis lives. Actually it has never been so full of flowers. June, Weird bug sighted on it and flung that green, wormy thing into the trash. July, more bugs eating. Tried a baking soda

solution, and it seems to have spoiled their appetite. August, Bug free
and brimming with bountiful buds.

As part of *Shovel It: Nature's Health Plan*, get a book in which you want to do more than just make notes of that which prospers and that which dies. Blend the therapy of journaling for mind and soul with your gardening desires. Before you discount this garden job, listen to what Thalassa Cruso, gardener and author, writes: "Garden notebooks are instant nostalgia, and sometimes they can make you feel a little sad for times long since past. But if you keep them going and never let them become a series of faded relics, they will form a continuing microcosm of family history as well as an invaluable horticultural record. So do start one of your own, don't allow it to become a nuisance, and don't feel that it has to be fine literature; write in it when the spirit moves you. This way you will preserve for yourself, and perhaps for your children, a very pleasant account of how things were done by you and why."

Some gardeners, writers, therapists and others who journal use spiral tablets, found at bookstores, drugstores, grocery stores and the stationery shop. I recommend the journal as a private place in our too busy world to capture the feelings inside and to investigate them. You can buy journals that range from the really fancy leather ones to more simple versions.

I like inexpensive, yet attractive, spiral notebooks, the cheaper the better, and I usually find them on the sale shelves at the supermarket or big warehouse stores. While these notebooks are less expensive, you don't have to scrimp. Yes, friends have given me gardening journals and blank books that are too beautiful for words. However, they scare me. Not the friends, but the books. Why? In a leather-bound diary I'd feel compelled to jot only "important" ideas and thoughts. As you've realized, my gardening will never win prizes from Fine Gardening magazine, and if some garden authority came for a visit, I'd probably have a breakdown worrying about weeds and imperfections that are everywhere. No way will I tarnish a leather-bound (read: expensive) book with my gardening thoughts and the dirt that I've been known to sport beneath my fingernails. However, in a notebook with cartoon characters decorating the cover, I can be playful and childlike.

I can cook up harebrained gardening schemes with the best of them. Yes, one of those round-the-bend ideas recently came to me. For a few deliciously playful minutes, I concocted a magical plan to build a tree house where I'd move my office. Of course, somehow I'd have to buy and then plant a really big tree to support it all. Then I'd have to figure out how to get the DSL cabling up the tree, wire it for the coffee maker and create steps so Zippy, my Welsh terrier, could visit when it was time to play fetch. I'm sharing this so that when you create wild ideas for your garden, you'll know that I've been down a similar garden path. That's what our journals are for.

If you buy journals on the cheap, please don't scrimp on a pen. I prefer to write on paper that's smooth so that my fountain pen will glide over it. If you're still writing in your journal with a scratchy old pencil that the kids won't even use, *Shovel It* and get a pen worthy of your creative, nurturing ideas.

There's no right or wrong way to write in your garden journal. I especially enjoy reaching this point in a presentation or when I'm teaching this class. For emerging gardeners or those who have tried many times to become more green-thumbed (sometimes half of the participants), I urge participating in the journal writing part of *Shovel It* for a minimum of six weeks. Writing in a journal or any new habit, whether it's good or bad, takes six weeks to become established.

You may want to compare notes with others or share ideas and plans from your journal with spouses, co-workers, kids and friends. I don't recommend allowing others to read your journal. Never. Ever. As a matter of fact, I'd like to suggest you not read or edit the writing in your journal for the first six weeks. Doing so might stifle your creativity and may turn you off discovering why you're taking your healthy body and mind so seriously when there's so much else to do. (Because, of course, if you don't take care of yourself, no one else will. But you knew that answer, right?)

Allow the thoughts that appear in these pages to come from your heart and your brain. Initially, the time you spend with your journal might feel like a huge complaint session and may even have little to do with what's growing or dying or being shoveled. It could be you'll write the "he did this, she did that" stuff and then one day, out of the blue, will come a desire to write about the sumac that's threatening to turn screaming red. Suddenly you might want to document every day of that fall, with your hopes and dreams and the tree's leaves as a metaphor of the cycles of your life. You might discover a memory that has long been forgotten. You might want to sketch out a person whose behavior affected you in some way. You may want to use poetry to tell about your feelings of a time that changed your life.

In your journal be ready for the unexpected. That's the joy of journaling. You can keep your journal on your computer, but it's much nicer to use an old-fashioned, carry-able book. You may want to attach a pen, via a string, to the spiral binding, so you can jot notes as you walk around your garden. You'll definitely want to have it as you sketch and dream and record the activities in your backyard.

Spend five minutes to a half-hour a day writing in your garden journal. Many find that first thing in the morning is the best time to spend with a journal. Some do it at lunchtime at work or just before bed. I like to sit with it, make friends with it, and then scribble notes, produce a drawing or just know that it's close by.

As you start writing in your journal, you'll probably be surprised that you begin to remember experiences that seem to have been buried in your past. You may be shocked at how clearly you remember the incidents long forgotten or ideas that come from nowhere you can figure. Don't be surprised if, after writing in your journal for a few weeks, your dreams become more vivid and memories surface at the oddest times. This is healthy. Keep these thoughts in your journal. Do not struggle to make sense of them, just jot them down. The process itself is healing.

If there are areas needing to be pondered, do so in a gentle way. Gina, a woman in a gardening lecture told me how, by using her journal, she realized why she'd become a perfectionist about gardening. The trouble wasn't that everything always had to be perfect for her, no matter what, but that she couldn't relax in the garden. So instead of unwinding, she became more distraught when she looked at her yard. There was no joy to it, only work. I've visited and sat in her garden. It's a lovely, suburban retreat with the three P's, patio, pool and play equipment for the kids.

As Gina told the story, "One day as I was mowing the lawn, I stopped, rushed indoors to get my notebook and scribbled: Weeds everywhere."

Then she remembered. "Weeds everywhere" was hollered time and again by her father when she was a small child. Although disabled, he still gardened after an accident at the factory where he worked. In a wheelchair, he could no longer mow the lawn, which had been his Saturday morning ritual. After the accident he'd hired a string of neighborhood teenagers to mow the lawn to perfection and get out the weeds.

Gina shared that she asked her father, now in a retirement community and addicted to puttering in small flower beds, about the incident. "I was shocked. Dad only vaguely remembered this image," Gina said. "Rather, when I cornered him on it, he said, 'If you say I yelled, I probably did. I wasn't myself for a long time after that forklift crushed me. Trouble feeling like the man of the family, you know. Could've taken it out on the kids mowing the lawn. Did it hurt you, honey? I wasn't mad at you.'"

Would this woman have discovered why she hated weeds or other garden imperfections if it hadn't been for the journal? Rather than assume any answer, I think that Nature would have directed her toward this information another way. But you never know.

Use the gardening journal to record your thoughts, your garden's successes and the failures, too. Use it to investigate gardening stumbling blocks and as a place to be silly.

As an alternative to writing in a journal, document your garden with photos, and then create a scrapbook. We'll talk more about this in chapter 7. You need not be an expert with a camera, but create pictures that please you. Once again, as with a written garden journal, you need not share this. This is part of your secret to regaining health, relaxing and finding happiness in your garden.

> *Almost against my will, I began reading*
> *about rose care. I just couldn't help myself,*
> *sort of like driving past a really bad car*
> *accident and not being able to look*
> *away...Of course, I admitted none of this...*
> *—Meg Des Camp, Slug Tossing*

Here I stand, I cannot do otherwise.
—Martin Luther
(speech, Diet of Worms, 1521)

Start Where You Are

Let's say you've just moved into a condo. There's a great deck or balcony and maybe some grass. If you're feeling like you're living in a room with no decorations, no cozy extras and no touches of your own, you're right. So much potential can be intimidating. It must feel this way when an artist looks at a blank canvas. I feel this emotion when, as a writer, I stare at a blank computer screen awaiting the Muse. The steps to creating are all the same. You must begin.

You still need to start, even if you're looking at your yard in a new way, especially now that you've done the Garden Bubble and taken the Garden Personality Assessment. It could be that you love your garden but know it could be more of a therapeutic place or just be more fun. It's time for a change, but how? Where? You may have some more ideas after writing in your gardening journal, but there's still more to ponder.

Some folks think of gardening as possibilities waiting to happen. For others the opportunities are terrifying, overwhelming and a hurdle that's too tall to cross. Yes, there are responsibilities when you start with grass and cement, and they can be weighty. What if you plant something you hate? What if it doesn't do well? What if this? What if that? Well, what if?

Get a grip. Think about the seasons. Every year, Nature changes everything. Heads to tails, it goes. Winter comes, plants die and trees go dormant. Spring comes, some plants return. In summer, everything that's supposed to live (according to Nature's plan) thrives. In the fall, plants fade, go into hibernation and wait for winter. Your garden—this blank canvas—is going to change every day. You do not control Nature, nor should you ever think you can. This could be a scary thought, but why not, at least for the next few weeks, just flow with Nature. Shovel the idea of controlling the uncontrollable. It's not going to happen.

Have you ever noticed how quickly Nature takes over when humans turn their backs? Maybe you've seen it with your front lawn or back garden when you've been away on vacation. Everything's tidy when you pack the suitcases, but by the time you're shaking sand out of the kids clothing, the place has turned into a jungle. I saw that recently when an elderly neighbor passed on. Betty had a meadow garden, and she worked to keep it lovely. We often swapped gardening stories, traded seeds, seedlings and cheery hellos over her fence as Zippy and I hiked through the neighborhood. Barely a year after her passing, without Betty's vigilance weeds were waist-high, trees were shaggy and vines were covering the back porch.

Flow with nature and learn from her, too. Just read over the nifty tricks to getting free and nearly free plants, just in case you don't have a friend like Betty, because you needn't spend a wad for a beautiful garden.

Take advantage of gardening friends who are blessed with an overabundance of something you'd love to have. Just ask and you'll be given. Trust me on this. A few years ago, my dear friend Ellen gave me some clippings from her feverfew daisies. Thought by many to have medicinal qualities, this daisy-like flower spreads like wildfire in the temperate San Diego coastal climate. It's now everywhere. If it weren't so darned pretty, I might feel guilty since I've now helped spread feverfew through friends to more than five gardens. It seems everywhere a seed is sprinkled a plant shoots up. Have you had this experience? Why, just this morning, I saw a tiny one springing up between the cracks of the front sidewalk. Thank heavens there are no plant police to cite me for littering seeds.

Share, swap and barter for plants you want and need. You'll have a better garden, a more joyful spirit and make others smile. Nature will smile on you, too.

Clone your leftovers. It's not necessary to buy seeds or plants to have a garden. With avocado pits, the top of a pineapple and a sweet potato you can have a luscious garden with plants that won't cost you an extra penny. You'll need a sunny location, the pit, top or spud, small drinking glasses or jars, water, some toothpicks, an ice pick or a nail (to poke holes in the avocado pit if it's especially hard), potting soil and some pots. Kids and seniors especially love watching these cloned plants grow. My mother taught me these cloning tricks and I share them, as I hope you will. Cloning, although it wasn't called that then, was popular during the Great Depression. I'm told that sweet potatoes as kitchen windowsill plants were all the rage. Those who still remember the deprivation of that difficult time may especially love watching the long white roots sprout and the speed with which the leaves appear. Recently I encouraged a caregiver, Carla, to help her mother, an Alzheimer's patient, create one for old time's sake.

"Mother initially seemed confused with the sweet potato, which didn't actually surprise me, but as soon as I brought out the toothpicks and the glass filled with water, she went to work. She remembered what do to. I cannot tell you how glad this made my heart. Now every day, she's there at the windowsill. Together we talk about the plant. I've also heard her talk to George, the sweet potato's new name."

Here are the details: For an avocado tree, save the pit of an avocado, allow it to dry out. Poke three or four holes in the middle and insert toothpicks. Simply submerge the lower half of the pit in water. After a few weeks roots will emerge, and then a stem and leaves will appear at the top. You need to keep the container filled with water or your plant will dry out and die. At your convenience, or when the stem is about 6 inches tall, place the lower half of the pit and roots in potting soil, in a container that sits in a sunny spot. Make sure there are drain holes in the container, and water it when it's dry.

Sweet potato vines are beautiful, and you can decide if you want to plant the vine in your garden or just enjoy it as a houseplant. Place a blemish free (with no mold on it or deep cuts through the skin) sweet potato in a jar of water. You may need to support it with toothpicks as you did with the avocado pit. Place it on a sunny windowsill, and in a few days roots and leaves will appear. Add water as necessary to keep it level with the top of the jar. Later, plant the vine in a pot or directly in the garden for a sweet potato crop from your clone.

Tropical pineapple plants are fun to grow, regardless if you live in Maui or in Anchorage. Select a healthy-looking whole pineapple from the grocery store. You might want to ask the produce manager which pineapple is the freshest or to call you when a fresh shipment comes in. When the pineapple is ready to eat, save the bushy part for your new plant. This means you'll cut the pineapple about 1" below the leaf level. This is the core. Allow it to dry out so that it will not rot, and then plant the core in potting soil in a container that has drainage holes. Place your plant in a sunny location. Keep it moist. In a few weeks, you'll see new green leaves appear and roots will sprout beneath the soil. It takes about a year's time and if you're lucky you'll get more than an attractive plant, you'll be rewarded with a pineapple flower.

Seek out plant sales. Garden clubs, civic organizations and even horticultural units of your local college have plant sales. Watch for notices in the local newspaper about the events. You'll get some incredible buys and perhaps even have access to plants that are native to your area and not found in the local nurseries. Ask to be put on a mailing list or e-mailed about meetings. At the sales, you can snag some great buys on unusual and over-sized plants and flowers. Besides, you'll get an ear-full of advice at the same time. You might want to save up your gardening questions to consult with a homegrown gardening expert.

Consider joining a garden club or becoming a member at the national level. Gardener's websites are showing up on the Internet in abundance. Some have online gardening dictionaries or resources that supply help and information for the asking. You can find online chat groups and gardening newsletters that are helpful to learn more about vegetables and plants, flowers and exotics.

Save seeds and swap them with friends. Last year I stood amazed nearly every day at the poppies and calendulas shared by a dear friend, Laurie, who lives in the wilds, forty miles from Bend, Oregon. She'd sent seeds along with a card, and I simply scattered them without much thought. But then Nature did her magic and I gathered bouquet after bouquet from "Laurie's Garden."

Shrubs, trees and flowers have long life spans, and trust me, they'll grow and continue to grow. So think next year and the years after as you select and buy. If your budget is like mine, always in need of stretching when it comes to the garden, start with smaller plants. Let Nature and you nurture them, and voilá, they'll grow into huge ones. For instance, you can buy two huge pots of lavender and your herb garden will have a focal point instantly. But you'll come away with quite a bit less cash in your wallet. Select ten smaller lavender plants for half the price, knowing that next spring these will be huge, and you'll be at least $100 ahead. It's tempting to plant them shoulder-to-shoulder, so that flowers, herbs, bulbs and vegetables will cover all the bare space. But plants (and people) need elbow room. Allow for growth in yourself and your garden when collaborating with Nature.

Buy at a reputable nursery, garden center, a catalog or garden website. Yes, you may spend a bit extra, but you'll be better off than if you buy discounted, possibly unhealthy, plants. Grocery stores and warehouse stores sell plants at astoundingly low prices. However, sometimes their plants haven't gotten off to a strong start in life. Buying unhealthy plants or those past their prime might feel like an act of charity. On the contrary, the damage may be so deep that the plants will not respond even to your loving care. You might get it cheap, but you could be throwing your money away. Yes, I know they say the plants are guaranteed, but that guarantee may just not be worth the trouble.

Learn to propagate plants and grow them from seed. It's way cheaper to grow flowers and vegetables from seeds than to run down to the nursery for a full-sized plant. Further, if you're into unusual varieties, you may not be able to buy the plants you covet, but can get them from seed catalogs. If you're new to gardening, get helpful tips on growing plants from seeds from green-thumbed friends, or closely follow the instructions found on the packet of seeds.

Love never fails.
—J Corinthians, 13:8

Lord, give me the courage
and tenacity of a weed.
—Karel Capek,
The Gardener's Year, 1929

Gardens Galore

The gardens that you'll unearth in this section are meant to spur your imagination. They are suggestions. You are in charge and will get to call the shots. You'll make the decisions and the mistakes as to what's best for you at this moment. Your ideas will change. Stuff that looks perfect in someone else's yard may end up at the business end of your shovel. It's rather like your neighbor's lifestyle, spouse's fitness program or a colleague's retirement plan. Might seem like it could solve all your problems, but simply doesn't feel right.

Read over the descriptions and draw ideas. Sometimes a feature can be transplanted from one garden style (where it might look delightful), and it becomes a focal point in another. It's perfectly fine to mix and match gardens. I have a rose garden, a tropical area, and when I stretch my imagination, there's a meadow.

My garden is a comical and curious collection of plants and flowers with country-style artwork. There are primitively painted birdhouses, which are primitive because I painted them. There are street signs and sculptures tucked in unexpected places. If I were hard pressed and had to put a title on the garden, whimsical would be it. It's a fun collection of design styles. It's always changing and never perfect, but perfect for continuing therapy for me. That's what your garden should be.

If the truth were told, I actually like the idea that there's always work to be done in my garden, real, physical, muscle-burning work. I couldn't find happiness in a garden where there were no weeds to pull, no bushes that needed trimming and no spent flowers and roses to clip. Anytime and any day, I can walk out in my garden and find something that's past due to be done. Rather than make me crazy, it allows me a release from my career and family obligations for precious moments to sense Nature and have a short chat with her.

A shrub never whines, "Just a few more minutes." A rose bush never snips at you with, "I'll do it later." And if you've ever heard anything rude coming from a smart-mouthed maple, you didn't hear the story from me. Trimming, weeding, shoveling, nurturing, hauling and mowing are physical, spiritual and emotional labors that balance my busy life. I need them as much as sleep, love and food.

Let me share a story. June Ann, Fred and their three kids, who live outside Cleveland, have a backyard of play equipment, including a trampoline. It's a kids' bliss factory. Fred talked about how he used to cringe when he looked out at the swings and sand piles. He dreamed of a formal garden. "After college I visited some of the famous gardens in Europe, and I've never forgotten them." Of course plastic pools and perfectly sheared hedges don't mesh, and for the longest time, Fred thought he would have to swallow his dreams. As their jobs became more intense, the couple knew they needed the therapy of their own gardening projects.

Now on the east and west sides of their home, in an area once just a "pass between" from the street to the jungle gyms, are those manicured hedges and rows of orderly annuals. No, it's not a garden that will vie for status with Versailles, but it is filled with quiet shades of greens, grays, blues and a dusting of pink and white. The sidewalk is wide enough for kids to run on and sail through on their bikes and skateboards. Fred and June Ann can putter, primp and trim. They're near the kids, yet can feel a world away. I found it interesting that they garden both together and alone, as if there are times when they want to think through problems and everyday hassles and other times when they need to share.

Gardening and healthy relationships have much in common: Both take a commitment, both take time and both take work.

"Someday we'll renovate the backyard and create an English garden, complete with a fountain as the axis, but for now, the kids need a safe place to be kids—and that's our garden. We can wait until they don't need this play area," June Ann said recently as we watched the kids and dogs run in circles around the water slide.

Let your heart and your head decide on the garden style. Also be aware that your style might be wild—with a bit of this and more of that. Wild, unkempt, always needing attention can be a style that works for you. Does for me.

If you want to kick it up a notch and create something unique, go directly to a bookstore, a big one, a gardening bookstore if you can find one. These are filled with books that are devoted entirely to one single type of gardening from shade gardens to herb gardens to how to mow your lawn to rival the one at Yankee Stadium.

The gardens presented here are a jumping off point to get you started on a therapeutic journey.

In each description you'll discover health and wellness tips to make this style of garden respond to your needs and your specific therapy. I've also assigned "attention level" ratings to give the scoop on how much time you'll need to care for the garden once everything is established.

H = high. Expect to put in at least 10 or more hours a week keeping this garden in apple-pie order.

A = average. This garden can be tended at odd times, or in the evenings and on weekends. It will require at least four or more hours of work each week, and more during specific seasons. It can be left alone for weeks, when it's being watered, and still look okay.

L = low and little work once it's established. We're not talking about the magic of going on an eight-week holiday and finding the garden in a bang-up beautiful perfect shape on your return. Instead "L" means that with an hour or two each weekend, you can still enjoy being outdoors, have the therapy of relaxation among Nature's flora but not become a flora slave.

Keep in mind that you can mix the ratings. You may want a low-maintenance garden, but have lots of potted plants that need watering every single solitary day. Use the guides as a reality check as you begin the serious work of gardening as therapy.

If what you put in a garden makes you happy, then the garden will be a happy place to sit, read, pray and enjoy.

Life is mostly froth and bubble,
Two things stand like stone,
Kindness in another's trouble,
courage in your own.
—Adam Lindsay Gordon,
English Poet

The garden: a thing of beauty
and a job forever.
—Anonymous

Garden Styles That Beg For You

Collector Gardens: Rated "H," these are the ones for passionate and determined gardeners with flexibility with finances and time. Trust me, I know you're out there and you're consumed with dedication for the collector garden. If you're delirious over daylilies, then you'll be willing to devote every inch of garden space for this type. Ditto with iris, cacti, dahlias or you name it, and there's been a collector who is wallowing in the passion of it all.

For health and therapy value, the collector garden is the right choice when flowers, vegetables or exotic plants mean only one variety to you. Besides, if you're gaga over gloxinia, you'd probably neglect all the other flowers in the garden anyhow, so why not focus your efforts?

The collector garden can be as formal or casual as you choose. You can design hardscape to give a backdrop to the drama of one variety. Collector gardens work well blended with Formal Gardens and with your collection displayed in raised beds.

Adding sculpture or art fulfills your sense of adventure. Add an oversized fountain or a delicate sundial as a focal point. While the garden style might feel too confined for those who seek an outlet for a wide range of nurturing needs, it can be a showplace, a singular haven or a private sanctuary for the senses because the variety is limited.

If you're considering a collector garden, most flowers have a limited bloom season. Will you still love it when the hollyhocks have faded and there's nothing there to replace their beauty? You'll need to have a year-round plan for this garden by staggering the plantings, or have the hardscape designed in an inviting way to make your garden enjoyable 12 months a year.

Formal Gardens: Rated "H," formal gardens are reminiscent of a movie set in England, especially the Victorian or Regency periods. They conjure up images straight from an historical romance novel.

As gardening's grande dame Penelope Hobhouse says in *The Country Gardener*, "The eighteenth-century view of the garden was that it should lead the observer to the enjoyment of the aesthetic sentiments of regularity and order, proportion, color and utility, and, furthermore, be capable of arousing feelings of grandeur, gaiety, sadness, wildness, domesticity, surprise and secrecy." Phew. That's a big job for a garden, and the goal of many who decide that a formal garden is the alpha and omega of their happiness, their peace and their ultimate therapy.

Seriously, if you're a romantic or think you should have been born in another time and want to feel needed (because the formal garden requires attention by the boatload), then you'll find therapy here. The formal garden forces you into servitude.

The formal garden demands strong symmetry and careful placement of flowers, plants and (sometimes) raised beds. There are focal points such as fountains or birdbaths as water features, and everything is built around the axis that is in the center of the formal garden. Evergreen hedges are sheared and line the pathways, and colors lean to the green palate, subtle and manicured. This is where the high attention level comes in, and unless you enjoy the work or can find pleasure paying a crew of gardeners, this garden means huge tasks to maintain. The formal garden works best with a formal architectural style home, such as a two-story colonial or Federal style, or a Mediterranean villa. Sure, you can still have a sprawling formal garden surrounding a California ranch house, but it won't have that same "wow" effect.

Hanging Gardens: Rated "A" or "L," depending on plant choice, the hanging garden is a dream come true for gardeners who want the therapy of planting, primping and pruning without the work of a full-blown garden. This is the right choice for those gardeners who cannot comfortably bend down to the soil to plant, cultivate and weed. Balconies, patios and apartment-sized gardens are perfect for hanging gardens (and mobile ones, as you'll soon see).

Hanging containers need special attention and for most plantings, daily watering. Soil must never dry out. Containers can be suspended from the roof, tree limbs or brackets mounted on walls and posts. A hanging garden may be the only choice for those with limited gardening possibilities. It's the answer, too, if you need a dose of instant therapy. Hanging gardens can bring Nature's pleasure to even the simplest patio or balcony and, therefore, pleasure to the gardener.

Annuals are the plants of choice for hanging gardens, which means in summer you could have impatiens for the intense colors and then fill the same planters with rust-colored or magenta mums in the fall. The plants you select will depend on how much sunshine is available in your garden area. A few plants that do well with just two to three hours of sun are begonia, lobelia and fuchsia. For a sunny spot, lantana, sweet alyssum, geraniums and petunias are good choices. In the shade, ferns do well. Lots of vegetables do well in hanging containers, especially tomatoes.

Low-maintenance, Low-water Garden: "L" is the rating for this therapy garden, with a warning. It takes planning and careful selection of plants to make the low-maintenance, low-water garden work.

This no-frills but still beautiful garden works for those who travel a lot, spend summers out of the area or live in the desert. To select the appropriate plants to make it worry-free, talk with the agricultural extension office in your area or with your city's water department. Ask a specialist at your garden center for more information, and check out the books specifically addressing the plants native to your region.

If it's restful therapy you want from this garden, then select fascinating rocks and sculptures as focal points, and use native or drought-tolerant plants as accents.

Mediterranean Garden: Rated "A" that could lean toward "H," the Mediterranean garden isn't as fussy and proper as the formal garden, but makes a grand statement, nonetheless. Think of *A Year in Provence or Under the Tuscan Sun* and you'll "see" this garden type.

The good news is that even in cold weather climates, you can have a Mediterranean-style garden. Yes, the garden blends with homes in the west. Craftsman style and Mission style homes, especially those of stucco, complement the type, too.

Rather than a lawn, most Mediterranean-style gardens have gravel or stone pathways, with berms and swales, and a multiple array of colors and textures. Walls are covered with vines, and terra cotta planters are overflowing with herbs and edibles. Fire-engine-red geraniums, pink coneflowers and bright white roses accentuate the contrast and texture of the gravel and walls. If your idea of therapy is puttering among the herbs and flowers and fragrant plants, you'll want to investigate this garden. Most Mediterranean gardens use herbs contrasted with flowers and share some aromatherapy with every visit. They're especially restful if you're seeking a retreat from a hectic world.

Mobile Gardens: The rating "L" is appropriate here because you can make a mobile garden anything you want at any time. "Move it, don't lose it" should be the slogan for those with dreams of a garden, yet unable to plant in the ground on which they live, like apartment dwellers and other folks who rent.

Consider the size and weight of container plants as a criteria for mobility. A potted palm might look perfect on your balcony but pose a threat to the building's structure when it gets taller. Many mobile gardeners, including windowsill gardeners, go in for smaller potted plants, orchids and tropical plants, which can also be brought inside during winter. The mobile garden may be the only therapy choice for those who don't own a home but still want to enjoy the positive effects of therapy.

Here's a trick to help with mobility for your big pots of plants: Fill the lower half of pots or barrels with Styrofoam "popcorn" (yes, a use for that white, sticky stuff), add a half inch of gravel and fill the top half with potting soil. This will cut the weight down and make it more mobile.

With all mobile gardens, daily watering is an absolute necessity. Ignore this need and you'll have plenty to shovel because the plants require a commitment.

Monochromatic Gardens: Rated "A" because you'll need to give this one attention throughout the year. The Monochromatic garden is fun. Some of us are nuts for pink, orange, blue or yellow flowers and design a garden around a single color. With green as the backdrop, it's the best thing since pockets.

If you want to feel drenched in your favorite color, then a Monochromatic Garden will be good therapy. One year, I did my front flower beds in white, another year it was yellow and the third year was blue. It's fun to plan and change the color and a challenge, too, to find related colors in flowering plants and bushes.

All-white gardens have a crisp and clean, fresh appeal. Now add Baby's Breath and a climbing white rose like French Lace to make it feel frilly. Light colors produce a feeling of child-like innocence. Blues are cooling and especially soothing, and you can achieve this with delphiniums, bachelor buttons and blue flax. Pinks are cheery and playful and abound in the flower world. Lavenders seem to invite you to unwind, especially when mixed with mauve like Echinacea purpurea and salvia. While not strictly monochromatic, a range of colors from pale pink to scarlet, the pinks of cosmos to salmon-color snapdragons, could work well. Be sure to use the lighter colors near the front and the more startling ones in the rear.

If you want to try out the therapeutic value of a monochromatic garden, arrange it all in a container—or do containers with flowers that are in the same tones. The effect is striking. We'll talk more about one-color gardens and what they say about the gardener in chapter 4.

> To create a garden is to search for a better
> world. In our effort to improve nature, we
> are guided by a vision of paradise.
> Whether the result is a horticultural
> masterpiece or only a modest vegetable
> patch, it is based on the expectation of a
> glorious future. This hope for the future is at
> the heart of all gardens.
> —Marina Schinz, Visions of Paradise.

Oriental Gardens: Rated "H" if you want the Oriental garden to be perfect, yet the therapeutic effect is evident here for all your senses. Think serenity. Peace. Water. Wind. Gravel pathways and tranquil fishponds with speckled koi gliding through the water. You may have decided this garden style could eradicate all your stress, yet the Oriental garden is high on upkeep, so it can produce plenty of worry. Here everything has symbolism, from the contours of the walkways to the height of the trees. And it's manicured. This isn't the style if you want to get out and putter, plant and change. If you want cut flowers, pass on this style.

If you prefer solitude and peace in its most delicious form, enjoy pondering life, praying and meditating outdoors and are looking for a connection of a lush exotic feel, then the Oriental garden is the perfect therapy for you. Green, a color that's known to help us relax and rekindle our energy levels, is the focal color of the Oriental garden. Structures are made of bamboo, wood or stone. Typically, there's a water feature or a dry riverbed. Colors come from cherry trees, green foliage, such as the Japanese cryptomeria and hemlock, and the blue/greens in juniper, dwarf spruce and pine. A few azaleas can mix in well, but don't even think about having them in cheery borders. In the fall, maples produce the accent colors. This is a high-maintenance garden, yet many find solace working in the tranquillity of the Oriental garden. This garden works best with contemporary architectural styles.

> Gardens are the result of a collaboration
> between art and nature.
> —Penelope Hobhouse, Garden Style

Raised Gardens: The attention level rating is "L" here, but of course, if you're really obsessive, you can fuss over the raised beds, too. Raised gardens are enclosed areas surrounded by wood (landscapers recommend treated redwood), stone or brick. With a wooden or stone ledge around the bed, one can sit comfortably while working on the garden. If the bed is knee high, physically challenged gardeners can work in the soil while sitting in a wheelchair.

Because the soil in raised beds can be improved and the plants and flowers maintained more easily, gardeners looking for therapy should find it satisfying. Raised beds are easy to work on and can look tidy with less attention. If you love the wild meadow look or want a bit of chaos for the senses, this isn't the right therapy garden style for you.

For ease, raised beds should be no wider than three feet if the bed is accessible only from one side, no more than six feet if it can be worked from both sides.

Many people prefer raised beds because you can have control of the soil and the maintenance is easier. Raised gardens can have a formal look that's symmetrical and work well as part of an English garden, or an informal look when they are used for vegetables.

Raised beds are the choice if your house was recently built or if you live in an area where soil has been depleted from over use. With raised beds you can add topsoil, compost and nutrients to produce the best vegetables or the biggest roses this side of heaven.

Rose Gardens: "A" is the rating for rose garden because they do need regular watering, feeding and looking after. Contrary to popular conception, a rose is not the fussy prima donna of the flower world. She's gotten a bad rap. But she does need some looking after to provide you with heavenly displays for months.

The rose is the most popular flower in America because of the recurrent blooms and varieties suited for all climate areas. If you're attracted to the rose but believe that it won't work for you, and you can afford one bush, purchase a specimen to see what happens. Really, they're a snap to grow. As you pick varieties, especially if you're new to gardening as part of Nature's Health Plan, look past the prissy and pretty faces of the roses you see in catalogs and online. Rather, select varieties that are disease resistant, hardy and fragrant. There are old roses, climbing roses, miniatures and huge bush roses. There is a rose that's right for every garden and container and works well with all architectural style homes.

Tip for roses: Roses loved being planted in the ground. And they're less fussy if you do. However, they can live a long, happy life in containers. The advice here: Never allow the containers to dry out—ever—or the rose will not do well. Sure, it might look okay for a year or so, but roses need a constant source of water to thrive.

Rustic and Naturalized Gardens: Rated "L" because of the easier-than-normal upkeep, the rustic garden does have a plan and takes some attention, especially in the spring when flowers tend to cascade over everything. Like the whimsical garden, the rustic one is out of control and loving it.

The rustic garden is casual, playful and surprising. With the naturalized variety, native plants seem to take over and control the mood. If your perfect therapeutic encounter includes rough grasses, graveled pathways, trees and plants similar to those seen in surrounding open areas, then this garden will work for you. It doesn't happen without attention. Because most gardens must be confined, why not use native plants that will work in your garden without taking over? For instance, goldenrod has lovely yellow flowers and grows like a weed in many areas. But for those folks who are highly allergic, adding this native to the rustic garden would be a nightmare.

Scent Garden: "A" is the rating for the scent garden, although after a year's worth of gardening, you'll probably have less to consume you. Initially, this garden takes time and attention, but if you're addicted to fragrance, you must have at least one part of your therapy dedicated to aromatic flowers, herbs and trees. Scent gardens work well in containers and in hanging pots, too.

The scent garden is usually filled with flowers and herbs, like the scented geranium and scads of rosemary creeping over walls. It has a rather wild look, since these plants tend to sprawl. If your idea of great therapy is breathing copious amounts of natural perfume, maybe mixed with a hint of mint, then you must take time to create a scent garden. They do take planning, especially if you want it scent-filled year round.

When selecting flowers and herbs, be sure to plant those you'll want to use in sachets and potpourri. Fragrant roses, like Mr. Lincoln and Cecile Brunner, and herbs such as rosemary and thyme, are especially nice in sachets. You'll feel like the ultimate creative gardener when you give these bundles tied with ribbons to special friends.

To make extremely inexpensive sachets, place about one-half cup of dried, scented floral mixture in a coffee filter (like you use for the coffee maker). Gather the edges of the paper and tie with a pretty ribbon. Great for inside the lingerie drawer.

> To be rooted is perhaps the most important
> and least recognized need of the human soul.
> —Simone Weil, The Need for Roots

Tropical Gardens: Rated "H" for those in cold or dry climates and "L" for those who live in frost-free, high humidity areas of the planet. Walk into a tropical garden, and you're in the jungle. Palms, bromeliads, orchids, ferns, cape honeysuckle, hibiscus and passion fruit vines cluster and clutter the landscape. Paths look like they belong when made of bark, gravel, brick or flagstone. Shade comes from palms and covered patios or shade cloths.

Most tropical gardens have water features and cascading ponds, some water plants and plenty of branching greenery that sways in the breeze. Think Hawaii, Mexico and Florida. Breathe in the scent of flowering ginger and you'll have a clear tropical garden picture.

If you fantasize about a tropical vacation or lifestyle, then you owe it to yourself to have a tropical garden for therapy (a mobile one if you live in an apartment or cool regions). Remember, you can produce the same soothing, trade wind breeze therapy by having just one small area of your garden as a tropical spot.

This garden style works best in a contemporary setting and may be too much in contrast to Victorian, Colonial, Federal or Mission style architecture.

Whimsical garden: Rated "L" because it can be anything you want at any time. The whimsical garden is designed to tickle your fancy and simply not make sense. This garden is magical, unruly, a bit messy and always changing. If you mingle with stodgy gardeners (those who must have everything in the best spot or they get the vapors), then you'll probably be chided for having a whimsical garden.

On the other hand, if you simply love fun things that make you chuckle at their sight, this garden style needs to be part of your health plan. If your day is structured, one colossal timetable, then the whimsical garden and you will thrive. The whimsical garden is the outlet to promote sanity.

In the whimsical garden you may find everything from totem poles to waterfalls, wrought iron sculptures and wooden signs that might say, "Garden Tours 5 Cents." In the whimsical garden, you might see a rusty bucket or a claw foot bathtub stuffed with Crassula falcata propeller plant or Echeveria elegans, commonly known as hen and chicks. There could be a wheelbarrow loaded with kale, cabbage, garlic, tomatoes, carnations, potatoes, daffodils and green pepper plants. If it's fanciful, capricious, weird and a little bit wacky, it fits in this garden style of anything goes.

This garden's joy is that it laughs at itself, and as your therapy, you must be willing to do so, too. With no rules and no requirements to make everything perfect the therapeutic effect is emancipating.

Keep in mind that this garden style never looks finished. It's the garden style of choice for lots of us because it goes with any architectural style and it's fun.

In the whimsical garden, you'll want to include plenty of flowers and bulbs for a long, staggered blooming season. This means you'll want annuals to change as the seasons do, along with a solid foundation of perennials, shrubs and trees. While the colors for the formal garden are subdued, the whimsical garden wants to shock and surprise you. If you select this garden variety, think of year-round beauty, and then forget the rules.

Wild Meadow Garden: "L" is the rating for this untamed child of gardens. However, this isn't everyone's mecca of garden delight. Some might compare it to a weed patch or worse.

With a meadow, the more sprawling and out of control, the better. If you have fond memories of frolicking in acres of flowers and butterflies and bumblebees, then you owe it to your therapy to plant a meadow. This is the garden to share with wildlife. Be sure to include a place to read, rest and meditate, and select flowers and bulbs that will naturalize (spread of their own accord) in your meadow. If you still want a meadow look but have a small garden, you can recreate a tiny version in large containers or raised beds. The huge wooden barrels sold at garden centers can be perfect for a portable meadow.

If "heartache" sounds exaggerated then
surely you have never gone to your garden
one rare morning in June to find that the
frost, without any perceptible motive, any
hope of personal gain, has quietly killed your
strawberry blossoms, tomatoes, lima and
green beans, corn, squash, cucumbers. A
brilliant sun is now smiling at this disaster
with an insensitive cheerfulness as out of
place as a funny story would be if someone
you loved had just died.
—Ruth Stout, How to Have a Green Thumb
Without an Aching Back

Some meadow advocates bristle at the mere mention of lawns. They advocate taking out ever-thirsty lawns and replacing them with meadow. They imply that it's a crime to have all that nonproductive area. But I take a middle-of-the-road approach because I like to walk barefoot on grass, have a picnic lunch on my lawn and play ball with my dog on this nonproductive area. Grass feels good.

Why not put up signs saying "Birds welcome." If you design your meadow with water, shade and shelter (in the form of bird or nesting houses), then wildlife will come. Birds need water and places to hang out, as in unclipped shrubs. We'll talk more about sharing your garden with birds in chapter 7; it's easier and more fun than you may think. Besides kids and seniors, those who are housebound find great joy and therapy from a bird-filled garden.

A planted wild meadow takes preparation. The most important job here is the selection of the best wildflower seeds for your area. Then you can't just let Nature control it, but must give the meadow regular periods of water and fertilizer. Even in this haphazard garden, you'll need to weed. Weeds which choke out the less hardy varieties and rob water from others are the reason most wild meadows fail. Many weeds spring forth in the first year of your meadow, and you'll need to identify which ones come out and which are there to stay.

To make your meadow a wholesome place for wild critters, do not use insecticides. Most birds eat spiders, worms and other insects, and by using bug killers you'll actually be hurting the birds you want.

You needn't go into the wild to find wildflower seeds, rather, you can buy them at most nurseries and through catalogs. You may need to bring in a load of rich topsoil if your ground is lacking. Dig in plenty of organic material, like composted leaves, to loosen and enrich the soil.

The meadow look is chaos. It's colors, textures, shapes and sizes. Meadows require full sun. If you like prim and perfect, you won't find much therapy here.

To get the most therapy out of the wild meadow, come to terms with the idea that at least two seasons of the year it will look dead (you can read that as resting, if you want). To lessen the uglies, bring in lawn chairs or a wooden bench to the meadow, perhaps a patio. Then when the meadow is less-than-lovely, you can create a mobile garden.

Soil: a type of dark mud in short supply
in the garden but readily found on paths,
patios, verandahs, clothing, boots,
and kids' feet.
—Anonymous

*The more I hear of Horticulture, the more I
like plain gardening.
—Julian R. Meade, author*

Draw It All:
Your Garden Job

On a piece of paper—copy or printer paper will do—draw a sketch of your yard. Now draw circles around the areas as you see them planted. This is your map—at least for now.

Some folks do this in a multi-stage plan, as the wallet or energy or time allows. Stage one might be to put in grass and a sprinkling system. Stage two might be to build raised flowerbeds along the wall at the back of the garden. Stage three could be to fill that raised bed with annuals.

Sketch different ways that you could design the landscape. Use various colored pens or crayons for the colors of the deck, the kids play area or the rose garden.

As you become a landscape designer, remember, Nature is in charge. Keep in mind the sun's direction and where you'll want to hang out. Put in a water feature, add a deck or flagstone path or set up a croquet court. Be wild and adventurous. Go for at least ten sketches, and yes, I know that's pushing your creativity, but that is the idea of this garden job. So after you've done several, lay them on a table or hang them on the wall.

Live with them for a few days and compare and modify as you go. Unless you're in a huge hurry, wait a week and see what feels right for you.

Divide the yard into gardening units, one for shade and the picnic table, another for the play area, putting green or croquet court. Why, you can add berms and swales, focal points and rocks and boulders to change the personality with texture.

You can plant shrubs or trailing vines along the property line to make a small garden feel larger. You can install a piece of garden art that will become (at least for a while) a focal point in the garden as the garden moves through development stages.

Need to hide or conceal part of the garden or want some privacy? Make or buy a screen of bamboo or palm fronds to shield a therapy area from a neighbor's view.

In the next chapter, we'll talk about intimate gardens designed just for you, but first, let's get down and dirty. It's time to talk about soil.

A few words on dirt: Should you call it dirt or soil? What's all the fuss, and what does it matter? For our use, here in *Shovel It*, we'll use the terms interchangeably. For horticulturists, there's a world of difference. Since you'll be hanging out with plant people, here's the scoop.

On the surface, dirt and soil are the same. Soil is alive. Good soil is constantly changing and nurturing the plants, vegetables and flowers that grow in it. On the other hand, dirt is dead. It cannot support life.

Good soil has bacteria (good bacteria), worms, animal manure, organic matter from dead plants and healthy natural chemicals such as nitrogen and fine-grained sand. Dirt has no or few nutrients. Possibly there are large rocks or stones in dirt.

Soil, on the other hand, can support life. It does, in a sense, breathe. The respiration of animals, bacteria and the fungi in the soil produces ten times more carbon dioxide each year than the amount of carbon dioxide released by all the things that humans do, including burning fossil fuels. When plants die, they return to further feed the soil. Additionally, good soil has humus (decomposing plant materials) in it. This makes the soil dark and crumbly. It gives it that delicious earthy smell.

If you wonder how healthy your soil is or if, in fact, you have dirt (using the scientific definition), then test it with one of the soil testing kits available at garden centers or through an Internet gardening store.

> A rose-tree stood near the entrance
> of the garden: the roses on it were white,
> but there were three gardeners at it,
> busily painting them red.
> —Lewis Carroll

Chapter 4

It's You. It's You.
It's Personal.

Of the seven deadly sins, surely it is pride
that most commonly afflicts the gardener.
— Michael Pollan, Second Nature

Can you imagine a garden designed on a Bible theme? Do you know that your favorite color can become a personality garden and shout that you're gaga for green or in love with lavender? Would you like to have a shelter for your soul? Are you aware that there are ways to enhance a garden by just switching the placement of plants and furniture?

These are concepts you may never have considered, yet at this juncture it shouldn't seem that wild at all. Even with your creativity bursting and gardening fingers itching, you may want to see how you can further personalize your garden.

As any gardener will tell you, it feels good to dig in the soil. Do many consider it a therapeutic tool? Not enough, even though the proof is included in medical journals and expounded by scientists and physicians.

Professor Diane Relf is a leading voice on horticultural therapies and a professor of horticulture at Virginia Tech. *In Horticulture: A Therapeutic Tool*, she tells how gardening has been prescribed as a curative tool for many of the illnesses of the body and mind, including those of the nervous system. She writes, "In 1768, Benjamin Rush maintained that digging in the soil had a curative effect on the mentally ill, and by 1806, hospitals in Spain were emphasizing the benefits of agricultural and horticultural activities to the mental patients. Dr. Gregory in North Scotland was reported to have gained fame in the early 1800s for curing insanity by compelling his patients to work on his farm." She continues to explain that at Pontiac State Hospital in Pontiac, Michigan (founded in 1878), farming and gardening have been long-standing and essential parts of the work-therapy program. Initially, the programs were to provide work and food production for those in institutions, yet when a therapeutic link was verified, the emphasis was shifted.

Today, mental health professionals are also recommending gardening as a therapeutic tool, perhaps someday a prescription will be written on a packet of seeds: Plant these, tend these, harvest these, and you'll feel better. Or, follow the directions and call me next season.

Give these theories thought as you personalize your garden with the suggestions included below.

Gardener's Lament
The things I sow somehow don't grow /
I'm sorely disenchanted; /
But, oh, what luck I have with stuff /
I never even planted.
—Anonymous

God almighty first planted a garden. And,
indeed, it is the purest of human pleasures.
—Francis Bacon

Your Sanctuary, Spirituall y Speaking

It's a haven, a refuge and a hideaway. The garden can be a harbor in the storms that brew for you, your children and extended family. Depending on your beliefs, you may make all or part of your garden into a sanctuary or a restorative shelter or retreat. Regardless of your budget or your gardening abilities, there's a plan to create a sanctuary that's right for you. The impossible becomes possible when Nature works through you.

You have lots of history behind your desire to create a shelter for your soul. You might do it as simply as adding a religious statue to the current garden, or selecting a St. Francis-style bird feeder with the arms stretched out for all the winged creatures. Recently when we were hiking in Ireland, I was drawn to the stone pillars and crosses celebrating early Christian enclaves, but reality surfaced when I thought about lugging one back to San Diego. Maybe next trip.

Gardens were used for curative, restorative purposes in Persia, Egypt, the Orient and throughout Europe long before and during the Middle Ages. Many of these gardens were secret and private within the walls of convents and monasteries. In these safe havens, refugees were soothed by the restful and health effects of the plants, flowers and herbs, many of which were used for medicinal healing. The vegetables and fruits were grown to nourish the body as well as the soul. St. Bernard of Clairvaux, France, talked about his garden. He wrote, "Within this enclosure, many and various trees, prolific with every sort of fruit, make a veritable grove, which…offers to those who are strolling about a spacious walk, and to those overcome with the heat, a sweet place for repose."

Should you want a sweet spot for collecting your thoughts, you're in good company. In the mid-twentieth century, Mary's Garden literature began to be collected and identified. Groups were formed to research the hundreds of flowers named in Medieval times as symbols of life, mysteries and privileges of the blessed Virgin Mary, Mother of Jesus.

The inspiration for the first public Mary Garden was at Angelus Tower of St. Joseph's Church, in the village of Woods Hole, on Cape Cod, Massachusetts, in the 1920s when some fifty Flowers of Our Lady were planted in this garden. In 1951, volunteers distributed kits called "Our Lady's Garden." The material included seeds, bulbs, plants and a leaflet about how tending one's own Mary Garden could be a prayerful, religious work of stewardship for God's flower riches and artistry, with devotion, praise, thanksgiving, meditation and commitment. Mary Gardens shortly became established at schools, parishes, burial plots, institutions, shrines and homes throughout the world.

Early public Mary Gardens were in Havana, Cuba, on the roof of the Ambos Mundos Hotel, and at the Manila Observatory in the Philippines. Today some of the better-known Mary Gardens are at Our Lady's National Shrines at Knock, Ireland; Akita, Japan; at the Artane Oratory of the Resurrection in Dublin; and in the cloister planting of Lincoln Cathedral in England. In addition to the mother garden in Woods Hole, there are Mary Gardens in Ohio, Pennsylvania, Maryland and Michigan.

Perhaps you'd like to create a religious garden, whether in soil or pots, to create a theme or to tell a Bible story. This might also be an idea for a Sunday school class to add to a church's landscape. It is an enticing idea for your own garden as well as having it become a haven for a weary spirit.

Many gardeners who enjoy creating a religious sanctuary make or buy signs inscribed with Bible verses to enrich the meditation process. A sign can be a simple affair, marking pen on plastic or a carved or engraved sculpture to enhance your private retreat. You might want to add some bells, angel sculptures, or even fairy lights (like those used during Christmas) to brighten a summer garden or make a twilight stroll enticing.

Here are some plants and herbs with their Bible reference to get you started. You'll find more information on this topic in the bibliography and on the Internet. I especially like the Biblical references to flowers, and while some horticultural historians select one variety, such as the lily, to reveal God's message, I believe all flowers speak to our souls, our hearts and our minds if we have the sense to listen.

Aloe (aloe vera): This healing substance was brought to care for Jesus' dead body. "Nicodemus, who had at first come to Jesus by night, also came, bringing a mixture of myrrh and aloes…" —John 19:39

Anemone (anemone coronaria): These "lilies of the field" call us to trust in Jesus. "And why do you worry about clothing? Consider the lilies of the field, how they grow; they neither toil nor spin, yet I tell you, even Solomon in all his glory was not clothed like one of these." —Matthew 6:28

Barley (hordeum vulgare): "There is a boy here who has five barley loaves and two fish. But what are they among so many people?" —John 6:9. Yet, as the verse proceeds, this little treasure was given to Jesus and it fed 5,000 people.

Beans: The bean reminds us to be filled with a hospitable temperament. "When David came to Mahanaim, Shobi…brought…beans and lentils…for David and the people to eat." —2 Samuel 17:27-29

Coriander (coriandrum sativum): God fed the people in the wilderness with manna. "Now the manna was like coriander seed…" —Numbers 11:7

Dill (anethum graveolens): "Woe to you, scribes and Pharisees, hypocrites! For you tithe mint, dill and cumin, and have neglected the weightier matters of the law: justice and mercy and faith…" —Matthew 23:23

Endive (cichorium endiva): People of faith are called to remember God's saving action in the Exodus by celebrating a seder meal each Passover. "In the second month on the fourteenth day, at twilight, they shall keep it; they shall eat it with unleavened bread and bitter herbs." —Numbers 9:11

Fig: The fig shows signs of hope. "Neither shall they learn war any more; but they shall all sit under their own vines and under their own fig trees, and no one shall make them afraid." —Micah 4:3-4

Flowers (violets, chrysanthemums, lilies, daisies, roses and all others): Flowers remind us that life is fragile, is worth celebrating and is a call for us to be humble. "Let the believer who is lowly boast in being raised up and right in being brought low, because the rich will disappear like a flower in the field." —James 1:9-10 "The grass withers, the flower fades; but the word of our God will stand forever." —Isaiah 40:8 "The flowers appear on the earth; the time of singing has come, and the voice of the turtledove is heard in our land." —Song of Solomon 2:12

Garlic (allium sativum) and vegetables: These remind us of how ancestors complained about the luxuries they lost as they followed God. "We remembered the fish we used to eat in Egypt…the cucumbers, the melons, the leeks, the onions, and the garlic…" —Numbers 11:5

Lentil (lens culinaris): Esau traded his blessing as the oldest son for a bowl of lentil soup. "Then Jacob gave Esau bread and lentil stew, and he ate and drank, and rose and went his way. Thus Esau despised his birthright." —Genesis 25:34. The lentil asks, Are we trading our birthright and God's blessings for earthly delights?

Mustard (brassica nigra): Mustard reminds us of our faith and the power of God. "If you have faith the size of a mustard seed, you will say to this mountain, 'Move from here to there,' and it will move; and nothing will be impossible." — Matthew 17:20

Not ready to turn the entire garden into an Old or New Testament theme park? Then consider adding Bible plants and herbs to your established beds. It is possible that you'll find the act of planting, watering, nurturing and harvesting to be a spiritual experience as you share the bounty with others.

Yes, your positive energy can be transferred to others who are in need of better health. In a study in the early 1960s by psychologist-researcher Bernard Grad, of Montreal's McGill University, it was explained that our moods can affect the things around us. He tested whether or not mental depression might produce a negative effect on the growth of plants. This concept has been dubbed "The Green Thumb Effect."

According to Larry Dossey in *Reinventing Medicine*, "This idea fits with the common belief that some people have green thumbs and that one's thoughts and emotional states may play a role in how vigorously plants grow." Grad's theory proved correct. When people who were depressed watered plants, the plants grew more slowly. When people with upbeat personalities held a bottle of water and then poured it on plants (in the same fashion as those who were depressed) the "upbeat" plants grew more rapidly and became healthier.

As the late humorist Erma Bombeck said, "Never go to a doctor whose office plants have died." Through mechanisms not yet explained by science or the medical community, this study and others show that physical objects may pick up the moods of humans, and emotions can positively or negatively affect inanimate objects. Ever wonder why someone's grass is greener? Might be all in the mind. And stretching this theory further, perhaps when you share your bounty, those who receive it will be positively affected.

I don't know whether nice people
tent to grow roses
or growing roses makes people nice.
—Roland A. Browne, Author

There can be no other occupation like
gardening in which, if you were to creep up
behind someone at their work, you would
find them smiling.
—Marabel Osler, author

Garden Escape

Okay, you're dreaming of Hawaii, the Rockies or Palm Springs, but your vacation budget has only enough for a night at Motel 6. What's a body to do? Create a vacation area that requires no passport, no reservations which must be made thirty days in advance, and best yet, you'll find no additional credit card charges come the end of the month. You can have a garden getaway in your own backyard.

Since the *Shovel It* method says we need to get rid of those things that distract or annoy us, within reason, it may be that you'll have to temper your enthusiasm and make only part of the garden a getaway. Let's say the kids really love the skateboard ramp. Don't make your choice be it's either them or you, but rather disguise the objectionable area with tall plants, a "wall" of sunflowers, a hedge of mock orange, a bamboo screen or trees in pots. Haul to the dump or pop in the trash can dead plants and shrubs. Have a professional remove structures or even trim or remove trees that interfere with your getaway's plan. Yes, I know that this is dangerous talk, but sometime and somewhere you may have to be drastic if trees and plants are stopping your gardening dreams.

Be realistic. Plan your plantings. Make them versatile and design your garden for more than one vacation or getaway. Keep an eye on your budget, and realize that the world will not end if you must wait to install a pool or to take one out or have a crew remove a forest of poison ivy or fill in a gaping gully. Sometimes good things take a bit longer.

As you ponder a garden getaway, give attention to the edges as well as focal points. A ground cover to blanket a hillside might give you a restful feel without the cost of planting a forest. If you select a ground cover with lush green or blue green growth, it can produce the effect of the ocean or a lake in the background. If you're dreaming of a getaway, you'll want to keep it as low in maintenance as possible, so when buying ground cover, get the details for your specific application.

Remove those things from your getaway that offend you in any way (again, keep the kids, spouse, dog, in-laws, and others that the law protects). You may want to go back to the Garden Bubble to figure out what would be perfect in your getaway. One gardener who lives in a rented home bought large palm trees in pots, had a handyperson create a cabana and installed a tranquil water garden in a shady area in the backyard of her Phoenix home. To make it feel tropical, she also installed misting equipment for the trees and the psyche.

Go wild with garden art or souvenirs. Want a saucy Latin vacation? Why not create a directional sign and inscribe Spanish place names on it. Why, you can install Japanese pagodas, English-garden arches or prop a toboggan up against a tree for a Nordic effect. Really now, this is your getaway and you run the show.

Collect travel brochures, flip through travel magazines and study pictures of your favorite vacation spot. See what features you can duplicate in your garden. Check out the sites via the Internet, or get some travel videos.

I'm not suggesting that you hire a dozen workers and import tons of rock, dirt and grass if you love the Rockies. But you can use boulders with plantings of columbine, moss and thyme between the rocks to catch a rocky feeling with plantings. Create the feeling of moving water with river rock that seems to flow in a pathway. Add juniper, hostas, ferns, spring flowering bulbs and a wooden bench. You may want to tuck in some American violets, too, but be warned, violets can take over. Yes, there are worse things in life than having a carpet of perfume flowers beneath your feet, but at least know what you're getting into before you plant. With these tips, you can be freeway close to work, but still have that "I'm lost in the woods" experience. You'll want to provide a thick layer of bark around plants and make sure all the areas have access to plenty of water.

Ornamental grasses, such as pampas and blue fescue, provide sensual whispers in the garden, and grasses often attract birds and butterflies. Grasses are heavy feeders, though, and even though they look trouble free, some can be prima donnas. Talk to a garden specialist to find those grasses that are low maintenance, so you needn't be a slave to your garden. Poplar and birch trees rustle in the wind and produce a relaxing sensation that anyone who ever has to drive a freeway will love coming home to. Add a wind chime and a birdbath for more stress-free vacation time.

If lounging poolside is your vacation of choice, include fragrant plants and flowers in your getaway. Most herbs thrive in pots but require regular attention and watering. Garden torches and candles add romance, when well tended by adults, and shells give a tropical touch.

Why not grow your own organic vegetables and fruits? Even in small gardens you can do this when you select dwarf varieties that do well in containers. Imagine the next time you're sunning and get thirsty, simply reaching out and picking some homegrown lemons for lemonade. Grow some strawberries in a whiskey barrel and you can pop a few in your mouth as you settle in the sun with the latest best seller.

The best part of your garden getaway is that you can change it often by using potted and container plants whether you're gardening on forty acres or a balcony. Annuals work especially well if you want change, and your garden center will stock varieties that work for your area. Remember, bulbs are nearly foolproof. They're little workhorses of the horticultural world and hang in with you to give years of seasonal pleasure even if you've never had luck with anything green.

> I have spread my dreams under your feet;
> Tread softly, because you tread
> on my dreams.
> —William Butler Yeats,
> He Wishes for the Clothes of Heaven.

Flowers always make people better,
happier, and more helpful;
they are sunshine,
food and medicine to the soul.
—Luther Burbank

I Want Color,
and I Want It Now

If you've ever walked through a nursery or coveted a friend's garden that's in full bloom, you may have said these words: I want color. Color is everything to gardeners. We look at color to determine the health of leaves and the ripeness of fruit and vegetables. We look at color to blend with surroundings when we want a special mood for the garden. We often dress in like tones and have personal signature colors.

When planning and planting your garden, whether you're doing it in a pot on the windowsill or the entire acre of your backyard, a color-scape can refresh you, relax you or completely stir up your senses. Use color to find the right balance in Nature's Health Plan.

Basically, green blends with all of Nature's colors. Just look at any flower or plant. Red and yellow clash and jump out to shout, "Hey, you, in the garden, look at me. I'm here." For contrast, but not the screaming kind, place blues and yellows in the garden, such as the bluest lupine and brightest orange roses. White soothes and provides excellent contrast with other colors.

From the late 1800s through the 1930s, it was the rage to produce one-color gardens, especially white. Some people still crave an all-white flower bed, and home and garden magazines often idolize them. If you have the time and inclination, they're fun to produce.

A yellow garden stirs the soul and brain. If you want to add zip to a lackluster area, a yellow garden or a garden heavily colored with yellow, will do the trick. Check out the plants and flowers suitable to your area. Years ago, and alas, without my doing anything at all, a forest of sunflowers sprang up in our parking strip, between the sidewalk and street. Planted by birds (or God, depending on your philosophy), they were a showstopper. I've tried to replicate the effect and never succeeded. Really, I've tried. Once more, Nature just wanted to let me know that she is in charge.

The yellow-toned garden stimulates. Color therapists say that those people who prefer shades of yellow are creative and inventive, yet can be argumentative and outspoken. On the other hand, children seem drawn to yellow, and there continues to be something quirky and wonderful about that smiley, yellow happy face that you can see in a poppy or a Johnny Jump Up (known as a viola). Yellow flowers include Black-Eyed Susan (rudbeckia fulgida), buttercup (ranunculus lingua), daffodil (narcissus), evening primrose (oenothera biennis bienniel), Graham Thomas rose, sunflower (helianthus annuus), coreopsis (coreopsis verticillata) and yarrow (achillea).

The purple garden gives an impression of wealth, grandeur, majesty and opulence. This feeling harks back to the time when royalty chose the color as a symbol of distinction. Like a red one, purple gardens are exciting, and yet there's a feeling of mystery and contentment. There's power in purple. Color therapists and decorators say that "purple people" want to be known as unique, different and light-hearted, playful and cheerful, with an "I'm special" persona.

Purple really makes a statement as a border or surrounded by light-colored flowers and plants. In the garden you can have purple in allium (allium aflatunense), Brazilian verbena (verbena bonariensis perennial), lavenders, heliotrope (heliotropium arborescens), Japanese and Dutch iris, tulip and violets.

An all-green garden might be just the ticket if you 1) must deal with shade year round, and/or 2) prefer a restful, calming, quieting garden and/or 3) live in a hectic, crazy-making world. Green is the ultimate color of nature, and it comes in more shades than it's humanly possible to count. Green is the easiest color on the eyes, and those who prefer green say they like it because it's cleansing. Color therapists tell us that those who are "green people" are self-assured, modest yet powerful. Green symbolizes the color of renewal, eternal spring.

In the garden, green serves as the foundation for all colors and blends without any help from you or Nature. You can add more green with flowering tobacco (nicotiana), hosta, spurge (euphorbia characias), tassel flower (amaranthus caudatus) and zinnia, such as the variety called Envy. The St. Patrick rose is a yellow-ish green.

Red speaks to our hearts of Valentine's Day, of summer's warmth, of Christmas, and in the garden it can add a sense of "wow." There's never a neutral red. Even the smallest red flower or vegetable beckons with, "Well hello there, honey, and where have you been all my life?" A garden planted intensely in red may appear smaller, yet pulsate with energy. Color therapists say that those who prefer red gardens like to experience life at its fullest, want to have control and are typically extroverts (or extroverts at heart).

Red actually mixes well in the garden. If you've ever put a Mr. Lincoln rose (which will become more purple as it fades) next to a bundle of the Honor rose, you know what a knockout combination that can be. Add some soft gray leaves, however, say of Dusty Miller, and the entire bouquet tones down.

In the garden, you can have fun with red by adding bee balm (monarda), crocosmia, daylily (hemerocallis), red valerian (cretranthus rubber), scarlet sage (salvia splendens), tulip and zinnia (zinnia elegans' Scarlet Flame is as hot as it gets).

Blue is one of the all-time favorite colors and gardeners love it, too. It produces a feeling of tranquillity, and the color blue has been found to slow a pulse rate. It might be a perfect choice if you're creating a stress-reduction garden. Blue is often remembered as the Virgin Mary's mantle, and in Europe many ancient churches have blue ceilings.

In the garden, blue gives a feeling of coolness and freshness, but an all-blue garden could look somber, nearly lifeless. Gertrude Jekyll, the famous British gardener who fancied one-color gardens, chose to blend the blues for this reason. She found that a totally blue garden has a surprising effect. It made those who were optimistic feel blue. Great news about blue, however, is it makes gardens feel large. And surrounded by pinks, oranges, yellows and whites, the blues make the colors appear clearer.

Good blues include baby blue eyes (nemophilia menziesii), delphinium, agastache (Blue Fortune is a great choice), lobelia, hosta "flavocircinalis," artemisia and blue-shaded anemones.

Orange in a garden is upbeat, snappy, happy and robust. Think of pumpkins and falling leaves and an armful of marigolds. Orange has an invigorating effect. Let's say you want to give your energy level a lift, then pour on the orange. This works well, too, if the garden looks saggy and company is coming. It's sort of like putting on red nail polish or wearing a baseball cap. Color therapists say if you need a zap of energy or feel in the doldrums, then orange should be your remedy. Orange lights are sometimes used to counteract depression.

Orange in your garden can be overwhelming. Think of a full bed of marigolds, zinnias and the Tropicana rose. Why, you'd need dark glasses. Rather, consider orange as a focal point or an accent color. Orange works well in a dull, overlooked corner.

Imagine a pile of pumpkins and gourds stacked near the front door for a harvest display. A real eye catcher it would be.

Orange works well with blues and purples. Birds of Paradise naturally combine these colors and never clash. Orange-tones that are lighter, say apricot-colored roses, mix well. White enhances their mellowness and rusty mums bring out a homey feel.

Good orange choices are the California poppy (eschscholzia californica), daylily (hermerocallis fulva), Japanese primrose (primula japonica), marigold (Taget's "Deep Orange Lady" is a prime example of bright orange), nasturtium (which comes in lots of colors, but orange seems to be the most common), Oriental poppy (papaver orientale) and the torch lily (kniphofia triangularis).

Lavender is one of the top choices in garden colors, whether you're planting ornamental kale, the Angel Face rose or American violets. Blues, whites and yellows look brighter and greens richer next to this light, dusty purple shade. Lavender is the color of the goddess Diana and symbolizes honor, dignity and divinity. Color therapists say that those people who prefer lavender are self-contained and typically have a gentle, easy-going manner. Lavender gives a restful effect, and in the garden that can be inviting to the eye and the visitor.

It's a gardening fact that a small garden planted with many lavender-colored vegetables and flowers will appear to be larger.

In the garden, lavender is popular in bearded iris, butterfly bush (buddleia davidii), clary sage (salvia sclarea), clementis, crocus, lupine and meadow rue (thalictrum rochebruneanum's Lavender Mist is a good choice).

Pink gardens are happy gardens, or so they seem to the senses. People who prefer pink are upbeat, positive, typically have a contagious sense of humor and smile a lot. It's tough to feel down when you're wearing or surrounded by pink, so if you're looking for a way to make your garden more cheery, then pink it is. Besides, there are plenty of pink flowers and flowering plants to choose from.

Pink varies in intensity from pinkish magenta to tones on the orange side. Pink looks pinker when placed near white or blue, but may appear dull in a bouquet of red or yellows. Yet, vivid pinks are perfect with red and seem to bolster the colors. Many pink flowers are favorites of hummingbirds and butterflies, so if you're planning to attract birds and beneficial insects, pink is a great choice.

Good pink choices are weigela, rhododendrons, pink foxglove, and the Carefree Delight rose. Other pinks to make friends and family take notice include sweet pea (Jayne Amanda is a good choice), verbena (verbena sissinghurst), mallow (lavantera barnsley), cosmos (cosmos bipinnatus), aster (alma potschke) and veronica (rose shades).

White gardens were all the rage in the late 1800s and early 1900s, and every once in a while a magazine will tout the joys of a white garden. Personally, I love color too much to create a white garden. I've tried it and it's fun, and once in a while consider doing it again, just for the challenge. But honestly, I feel happiest surrounded by lots of colors.

White gardens are serenity itself. In the Renaissance, paintings of lilies and white roses depicted the Virgin Mary, and even today, white provokes a feeling of purity, innocence and peace. Color therapists say those who prefer white are conservative but often have incredible inner strength and untapped creative energies.

In the garden, white brightens the appearance of other flowers. It just perks things up, yet can cool things down, too. Many white flowers and flowering bushes have luscious fragrances, so if you enjoy a midnight stroll, a white garden (or one with lots of whites in it) could be the right tonic.

Whites to include in the garden could include anemone sylvestris, campanula, physostegia, the roses Iceberg and Honor, Queen Anne's lace (daucus carota), phlox (phlox paniculata), springtime's paperwhite narcissus, gardenia, calla lily (zantedeschia aethiopica), yarrow (achillea milleforium) and baby's breath (gypsophila paniculata).

Monotone gardens might seem too industrious to you, or perhaps too boring, but you can try the concept on a small scale in a planter box or pot. Experimenting with plants is fun. Imagine walking up to the front door of your home or condo and being greeted by a tub of fire-engine-red geraniums or a mini-meadow of sunny daffodils.

Can there be a love which does not make
demands on its object?
—Confucius

Sitting silently, / Doing nothing, / Spring comes, / And the grass grows by itself
—Osho, Discourses

Feng Shui
and Then Some

Feng means wind. Shui means water. Yet this ancient eastern art is more than the two components. It is thousands of years old and teaches the arrangements of the elements in our environment in order to attain luck, prosperity and health. Regardless of your belief or disbelief in the system, it's fun and helpful to have a working knowledge of these principles.

Pronounced "fung schway," this is a philosophy that creates an environment that today might be called ergonomic. Believers say it allows us to work efficiently, comfortably and successfully by following the patterns of nature. It assists people (for our purposes, gardeners) to avoid their worst location in any environment and select a more favorable one, or to adjust that worst location to make it a favorable one. I think of Feng Shui as an intuitive "this feels right" feeling for my garden.

In ancient China, the secrets of Feng Shui were closely guarded. Today there are books, courses, videos, tapes and personal consultants ready to help bring better balance to your home, office, life and garden. There are also self-appointed mystics that supposedly have special answers.

According to the experts at the American Feng Shui Institute, located in Monterey Park, California, there are no secrets, and a reading requires no guesswork. Practitioners who offer to fix or use occult "cures" to change the Feng Shui should be hired with one's eyes wide open.

Feng Shui is based on a set of theories and complex calculations derived from the ancient text, I-Ching. This text and the balance of the positive and the negative, or Yin and Yang, and the elements of fire, earth, metal, wood and water, provide information on the natural environment and magnetic field surrounding all things, according to experts in the art.

If you quickly scan books on Feng Shui, you will read about the "Ch'I". This is a word for positive energy. To alter an unhappy, unlucky or unpleasant garden, one increases the flow of Ch'I.

For the gardener who may not want to hire a Feng Shui expert, incorporating the essences of the art may include adding open, friendly spaces to the garden. That may include gently curved pathways, niches, seats, waterfalls, clear ponds (in which the sky can reflect), chimes or even flags and mirrors. Chimes are an easy addition and produce an almost instant feeling of calm. I love them. The chimes, which move with gentle wind, produce quiet tones to reassure the body and soul.

Planting in your garden can take on a whole new meaning when you consider the aspects of Feng Shui. Plants are assigned to the five Feng Shui categories of wood, fire, earth, metal and water. Woody plants are believed to increase movement. Fire plants, such as sunflower or daisy, symbolize beauty and humor. Earth plants, such as Clematis, embody stability and peace. Metal plants, like gray and blue ornamental grasses, provide a quality of strength and resilience. Water plants, including water lilies and water-loving plants such as summer asters, are for strong will and seriousness.

Here are the meanings of the elements and their application in our gardens.

Wood is considered the beginning of new life, and it is the originator of the five elements. A shrub or bushy plant sends out and pulls back Ch'I, which is a good thing since this means there's a flow of air in the garden. A dying or dead plant has no Ch'I and is actually a "Sha," or unsightly or bad influence. However, driftwood that is chosen for beauty can enhance Ch'I, and many rock gardens would feel out of place without it.

You can add this element with wooden arches, trellises and reed fencing to hide an unsightly area (such as trash cans or an alley).

Fire symbolizes energy, beauty and good humor. Instinctively we look at glowing zinnias and smile. That's the feeling of fire in our garden. Red plants and plants with red flowers add this energy. Red clay pots, a red mosaic, or red pavers on the pathway can increase this aspect. You can increase the energy, beauty and good humor of your garden with lights, mirrors and a favorite of mine, crystals or clear-colored stones around the base of plants or piled on a stack of rocks.

Earth brings stability to an unsettled world, much like a range of mountains makes us feel grounded. Boulders, rock gardens and rocks in a small windowsill display can have the same effect. You can also increase the stability of your experience in the garden with exposed dirt and thick layers of mulch. As you think of adding more of this element, Feng Shui experts suggest you design curvy or wavy pathways and perimeters of planters. Straight lines are considered negative.

Metal structures in the garden increase the friendliness and denote strength, stability and peace. You can incorporate metal in chimes, statuary or sculpture. But Feng Shui practitioners say that metal must not have sharp or pointed edges, and should be pleasing to the touch and to the eye. Metal is the most common use to remedy negative energies in the garden.

Water gives life to our world, and it enhances the life-giving elements of your garden. A water feature can help. You may want to install (or have installed) a brook, a waterfall, fishpond, fountain, birdbath or lily pond, all of which will reflect the daytime and night's sky.

In addition to these elements, practitioners of Feng Shui use a specially designed compass called a Lo-pan to decide where to place structures, features and objects. As you consider adding more Oriental harmony to your garden you may want to refer to a book on the topic and review the following.

Placing structures or objects in the north part of your garden can increase creativity, personal growth, new ideas, inspiration, prospects, career, music and the arts. The north is a good place for water elements and for metal tool sheds, ponds and whirlpools. Avoid stone, clay and exposed earth in the north of your garden.

The northeast part of your garden signifies knowledge, wisdom, meditation, reading, inner journeys, spiritual and intellectual growth and all of nature. The northeast is a good place for stone benches, rock gardens, repairing equipment, boulders, statuaries, brick and anything made of earth. You'll want the shapes to be low and flat here.

The east part of your garden is best for new life and growth, rebirth and rejuvenation, harmony, health, family life, nutrition and healing. This is a good area for fruit trees, vegetable gardens, herbs, play equipment, a place to stretch and do yoga or tai chi, and restful plants and trees. The shapes to enhance this area are columns and cylinders and metal garden furniture. Tools and white flowers should be avoided in this area.

The southeast part of your garden, according to Feng Shui practitioners, denotes wealth, abundance, material possessions and communication. The southeast can host a showy garden, filled to the brim with annuals, colorful vegetables and trees that flaunt chartreuse in the spring, deep emerald in the summer and a glowing rust montage in autumn. This may be a wonderful area for wooden furniture where you can sit and chat with friends, or relax with a juicy novel or the latest gardening book. The best shapes for the southeast are posts, cylinders and columns. It's suggested that one avoid metal garden accessories, metal wind chimes and metal furniture, tools and white flowers, including white flowering vegetables such as sugar peas and potatoes, in this part of the garden.

The south is the space of dreams, opportunity, aspirations, awards, fame, achievement, happiness, longevity and happy events. Here's where you'll want the barbeque, the fire pit, outdoor furniture for parties and places to sit or perhaps a spot to sneak a kiss or more. Try to keep surfaces low and flat here, and include ponds, waterfalls, or other water features such as a birdbath or a fountain.

The southwest is the garden area to encourage romance, marriage, motherhood, love relationships and partnerships. It's a good place for seating arrangements, perfect for intimate dinners for two, or spots for outdoor business meetings or gardening club brainstorming sessions. Here, too, you'll want to keep shapes flat and low to avoid obstructing the Ch'I. Avoid sharp edges in patio or deck furniture, fences, gates and structures, including statuary, in this area.

The west is the right place for children to play, to grow strong, and feel loved. It's the creativity zone, so if you're an artist, potter, crafter, weaver, poet or writer, you might want to use this area for a work or meditation spot. It's the area for harvest, healing, socializing and entertaining, too. The west is the area where you'll put the play equipment, plant a garden with medicinal herbs, and make a garden to enable those with sight, physical or emotional challenges to feel comfortable and convalesce. It's recommended that the shapes here be restricted to circles and arches, again, no sharp and pointed areas. Avoid barbeques, fire pits and outdoor stoves in the west.

The northwest is the area for fatherhood, helpful people, supporters, mentoring and interests outside of your home. In the northwest corner you might want to place statues of angels or deities, animals and cherubs. The northwest corner is the right place for wind chimes and elements that are affected by the wind. Here, too, make the shapes in circles and avoid using the northwest for barbeques, stoves and fire pits.

Feng Shui practitioners say there are ways to improve the harmony and Ch'I in your garden in addition to the techniques mentioned above. Here's how:

Mirrors: Place mirrors opposite an overbearing building or busy main road. This will also make an area feel larger and lighter.

Crystal balls or gazing balls are another ancient way to balance the Ch'I. They refract the light and disperse the Ch'I to a larger area.

Lights are symbolic of the sun and balance unfavorable areas of the garden (or, in fact, of a room). Place lights, candles or torches here to illuminate an area or to guide visitors on a pathway.

Chimes and bells: These connect with the wind and bring Ch'I into a garden. Hang near an entrance or window to moderate strong, negative energies.

Flowers, vegetables, shrubs and plants: These are symbols of nature and possess all the elements of Feng Shui. Healthy plants attract Ch'I and promote a feeling of beauty, growth and vitality. "Dead as a door nail" ones that you've not gotten around to shoveling out are said to produce negative energy. Those plants, shrubs and trees that naturally go into hibernation are not dead and do not produce negative energy.

Trees: All trees improve the Ch'I. They can protect, shield and balance a site. A tree behind the house, and seen from the street, is said to encourage good fortune for those who live there.

Fish ponds: A fish pond in a garden attracts Ch'I and promotes prosperity and good luck.

Swimming pools: These are best when they are oval or crescent-shaped. Rectangular pools with a corner pointing to the home are considered unfavorable and Feng Shui experts recommend using the above ways to alter and improve the Ch'I.

All that I have seen teaches me to trust the
Creator for all I have not seen.
—Ralph Waldo Emerson,
The Best of Ralph Waldo Emerson

Manifest plainness, Embrace simplicity,
Reduce selfishness, Have few desires
—Lao-Tzu (c. 6th century BC),
Tao Te Ching

Designing a Mini and a Mini-Mini Japanese Garden

Would you like to create a Japanese or Zen garden for therapy? It's really quite easy, and it could be just the prescription in Nature's Health Plan.

If you don't have access to a garden right now or want to design one for your desk or coffee table, the mini-mini garden will be perfect. The mini-mini garden works well for those who live in a group situation, such as at a care facility or hospital, and they make spectacular gifts. I keep mine on the kitchen windowsill and can redesign the patterns whenever I'm in the mood for therapy.

If you have the ability to create a Japanese garden in your backyard, the options can be expanded with just a bit of imagination.

The mini-mini Zen garden: You'll need a plain picture frame and a piece of plywood or sturdy cardboard the same dimensions as the outside of the frame. I like the looks of an 8 X 10 inch frame. You'll need from 2 to 4 cups of sand depending on the frame you use. You can get it at the shore or beach or buy builder's sand at the home improvement warehouse. I've even heard of gardeners using kitty litter before kitty ventures into it, but I prefer the finer texture of sand. If you go the kitty litter route, find the type with the smallest particles.

You'll also need some attractive pebbles, about five. Some people like to use crystals or colorful stones, pieces of beach glass or shells. The size of your pebbles is determined by your garden's dimensions, for instance with an 8 X 10, I like to use pebbles about the size of marbles. You'll also need a dowel, stick or even a fork to draw patterns in the sand. You may find a tiny toy rake that would work well, too.

Secure the plywood or cardboard to the frame with wood glue or adhesive and allow it to dry. Place the sand inside the frame and gently shake to distribute. Add the pebbles in a pleasing pattern and then draw more patterns in the sand. Don't like the first design? Take out the pebbles and draw new patterns.

The therapeutic part is planning the design, drawing the circles, squares, or curvy lines and replacing the pebbles. Make one and place it on the coffee or patio table before your next party, and your friends won't be able to stay away. By the way, kids and seniors really enjoy this project. It's rather like a therapeutic and natural Etch-A-Sketch.

The mini garden: Technically called a Tsubonina, a mini Japanese garden should be small enough to be enjoyed on a deck, balcony or small patio.

Select treated (also called rot-resistant) 2 X 4s to make a sturdy frame. On the bottom, secure 1 x 6 slats with one-inch gaps to allow water to drain. Staple landscape fabric to the bottom to hold in the soil. Add stones, shells and rocks to represent a shoreline. You may want to line up beach stones to represent a river of water flowing from the mountains (the larger rocks) to the ocean (the gravel you'll install). I like to use larger rocks in the back and smaller, beach stones near the edge. You may want to buy a stone with an indentation on a flat surface, to hold water.

The gravel is used to represent the ocean or lake in your mini-garden. Now place potting soil on the "shore" and select plants that you find attractive. Remember, they'll grow. I like using mossy ground covers, like baby tears, which will flow over the rocks. You can also put Oriental lanterns or small Japanese statues on the "shore."

Unlike the mini-mini garden above, you'll be committed to sprinkling or gently watering this garden, but it's a delightful way to invite Nature's Health Plan into a small space.

> Beginningless time and the present moment
> are the same...You have only to understand
> that time has no real existence
> —Huang-po,
> The Zen Teaching of Huang-po

Chapter 5

A Trowel, Some Sweat and A Better Body

*God is the friend of silence. Trees, flowers,
grass grow in silence. See the stars, moon
and sun, how they move in silence.*
—Mother Teresa,
For the Brotherhood of Man

Shovel It. Yes, go out and get a shovel and turn over the soil. It's good for you. Hey, it's okay to have fun in the dirt and get your hands, clothes and shoes muddy. This chapter is about playtime.

Now, don't look too serious. It's been proven that adults need playtime. Just between you and me, working in the garden is an acceptable way to have kid fun and not be considered infantile.

Even playing can be hard work, hard on the body, so in this chapter you'll find fitness activities, a stretch plan, some yoga to do outside when the weather's comfortable, and activities to relieve stress. Gardening has been proven to be an activity that reduces stress and is recommended by the American Heart Association and the American Medical Association for those patients concerned with heart health.

You need to play more, but don't just take my word for it. A shot of sheer fun is the antidote to everything from flagging creativity to Everest-size stress. According to psychiatrist Lenore Terr, M.D., authority on relaxation and author of *Beyond Love and Work: Why Adults Need to Play*, "Being playful allows us to feel less anxious and more in charge of our lives. Everything and anything is okay in play." She rates gardening high on the play list, and *Shovel It* fits right in with a recovery program. Dr. Terr says frequency matters more than duration. She believes it's important to play at least three times a week, and adds, "You'll get the benefits whether you do it for five minutes or two hours."

Not only do gardeners play outside in the open air, for many there are deeper connections to our need for fun. For instance, I've never done well in competitive sports, yet I will gladly match my hybrid tea roses to anyone's at the county fair. That's competition. Many play at gardening in order to nurture vegetables and plants. Some play for social reasons, as we might when we volunteer in a garden project at a care center or in an inner-city garden. Dr. Terr, a gardener herself, says, "The best single way to appreciate the benefits of adult play is to play oneself. A person's play can be solitary or mutual, imaginative or strictly present, athletic or stationary. Play benefits the individual and the individual's surroundings. One can feel it…Play feeds on play." All play researchers seem to agree that once a person knows how to play, it becomes easier to play under other circumstances and at other times of life. Anyone can begin taking a more playful approach when it's remembered that today is a good day to start.

A study published in the *Journal of the American Medical Association* suggested that moderate exercise, such as gardening a few times a week, may increase longevity (HealthNews, May 27, 1997). The study was performed with 40,000 post-menopausal women, who were followed for seven years. More activity, it was found, translated to greater health gains. The reduced mortality rates were usually due to lower rates of heart or respiratory disease. Another study published in the *New England Journal of Medicine* found that women who were physically active during their free time and at work were less likely to develop breast cancer. Researchers suggest that moderate levels of exercise reduce the levels of estrogen and progesterone in the body, reducing obesity and enhancing the immune system.

Further, the U.S. Center for Disease Control and the American College of Sports Medicine say that simple, everyday activities such as gardening can provide the exercise needed for a stronger heart and longer life. This study was published in 1994 and continues to gather positive evidence each year. Experts say any kind of exercise that can be done throughout the week is better than one workout of considerable length, and it's not necessary to sweat up a storm to achieve maximum health benefits. Moderate exercise helps strengthen the heart and keeps the metabolism up.

Since *Shovel It: Nature's Health Plan* is great for your mind, your body and your emotions, it just may be that physicians of the future will recommend, "Take this shovel, dig in the garden and then call me in the morning." That's what we'll focus on in this chapter: Fun and activity for all. So first off, let's see how those with special needs can join the fun and garden the *Shovel It* way.

Whatever befalls the Earth befalls the sons
of the Earth. Man does not weave the web
of life, he is merely a strand in it. Whatever
he does to the web he does to himself.
—Chief Seattle (1786–1866)

The first gathering of the garden in May of salads, radishes and herbs made me feel like a mother about her baby—how could anything so beautiful be mine. And this emotion of wonder filled me for each vegetable as it was gathered every year. There is nothing that is comparable to it, as satisfactory or as thrilling, as gathering the vegetables one has grown.
—Alice B. Toklas, author

Can-Do Gardens for All Needs

Gardens are special and can be created and enjoyed by everyone, especially people with special needs. I call them "can do" gardens, but in the language of horticultural therapists, these gardens are called "Enabling Gardens." According to the therapy and gardening experts at the Chicago Botanic Garden who work with a therapy gardening program, "An enabling garden is designed to make gardening accessible and enjoyable." That definition sounds like my perfect place in the sun or shade, winter and summer and all the times between.

An enabling garden requires some special thought, yet if you're about to create one, the bottom line is that whatever is included must work for you and your can-do garden.

Most enabling gardens are barrier free. They have structures that are designed to accommodate children, adults with disabilities and older adults.

You can make an enabling garden by creating raised beds designed so that the disabled gardener can reach the middle. If he or she cannot reach far, perhaps the garden will be in a barrel or large terra cotta pot. I suggest the use of containers with wheels in order to bring vegetable and flower gardens to the gardener.

Vertical gardens are the right solutions for the can-do gardener. Forget the rules you may have heard about flowers and plants needing to be grown in a certain way. Vertical gardening is quick, attractive and fun. Here's the scoop if you're thinking of having a garden "grow up" on vertical supports.

Are you aware that vegetables grown on a trellis produce more and the quality is often higher? When selecting plants for vertical gardens, choose ones that naturally vine, such as peas, berries, grapes and beans. Pumpkins and melons work well, too, and then there's my all-time favorite of cucumbers, especially the Japanese variety, that thrive in the vertical garden.

Because vertical plants bask in the sun all day, the yield is more abundant. You'll get better produce and bigger sun-loving flowers with a vertical crop. It's also easier to cultivate a vertical garden. Foliage in a vertical garden dries quickly, so there's less chance of infection from a fungal disease. Plus, vegetables grown off the ground are cleaner, less likely to be eaten by bugs and stay safe from root rot.

Lumber stores, home improvement and gardening centers and online gardening supply sources sell attractive and inexpensive trellises. For minimum upkeep, look at those made of plastic, such as PVC. If you have a fence that's in the sun all day, why not make your own trellis from wire, secured with nails or hooks. Bamboo stakes or tall tree limbs used as poles make great "tee-pee" vertical gardens. Imagine one built from sweet peas. You can buy poles at the home improvement store.

Vertical crops cast long shadows as the sun moves across the sky. If you're in a warm climate, this garden style can provide shade to vegetables or flowers that can't take the heat, such as lettuce and spinach. These vegetables love a cool afternoon.

With so many plants growing in a small area, keep soil rich with amendments and covered with mulch (to maintain a constant moisture level). You may need to water often and use a time-release fertilizer.

Vertical gardens can be tailored to individuals in wheelchairs, walkers or with joint or movement concerns. Gardening is made more comfortable with adequate seating and shade. Also important is paving that is wide, smooth and flat for walkers, canes, wheelchairs and for the visually challenged.

A gardening bench or even two is a wonderful part of the can-do garden. You'll want to buy or design one that's the right height for children or a gardener with limited mobility or who is using a walker.

Drip irrigation and soaker hoses, mulches and ground covers cut down on the time required to weed and water. Buckets and bins near the garden can store tools.

Here's a list of how to make gardening easier which incorporates some of my ideas with those used by designers of enabling gardens.

- ❀ Tie a cord around the handles of small tools to make retrieval easier should the tool be dropped.
- ❀ Use gloves to protect hands and help maintain a grip on the tools.
- ❀ Keep a large magnifying glass handy to see and identify small plants.
- ❀ Wear an apron especially designed for gardeners or carpenters, or a smock with large pockets to store seeds, clippers and small tools, even a seedling or two.
- ❀ Use a piece of lightweight plastic pipe to help sow seeds without bending over.

❀ Have handrails or hand grips in areas that might be slippery.

❀ Carry a whistle. A short blast will alert family or caregivers that the gardener needs assistance.

❀ Rig hanging gardens with a pulley system to lower them for watering and maintenance.

❀ Grow vertical gardens, even in containers.

❀ Choose plants that appeal to the sense of smell as well as sight. Scented gardens and fragrant flowers appeal to all gardeners.

❀ Create a theme garden, such as one referring to Bible verses, Native American plants and vegetables, or plants mentioned in the works of Shakespeare.

❀ Design a garden that's attractive to butterflies and birds.

❀ Create a garden with heritage vegetables, plants and flowers. "Heritage" in gardening terms refers to old-fashioned varieties that are no longer on the common market but were very popular in the early 1900s.

Those who don't understand Nature's Health Plan might believe that people with impaired vision cannot garden successfully. It's simply not so. Claude Monet, it's said, loved flowers as much as he loved painting, and while Monet eventually lost most of his vision, he never stopped gardening, nor did he stop painting. The most important characteristics for you, as a visually impaired gardener, are the readiness to ask for help (at times) and the willingness to plan and work in your garden. It's important to remember that all gardeners must abide by common sense and safety practices, especially with tools and sprays.

❀ Have your garden designed with wide, flat, smooth pathways and consider installing raised beds to make getting to your crops and flowers easier.

❀ A drip watering system or a hose and faucet near your garden will make the chore easier. You may want to get a system with a timer, too. Most plants, shrubs, vegetables and flowers thrive on one inch of water a week, and depending on your location and soil type, this may mean you'll need to water once a week, twice a week or not at all if you're enjoying a rainy season.

❀ Select the tools you need for the job to be done. If you have trouble carrying tools and using a cane or walker, a smock with a large pocket or a carpenter's tool belt can help out.

A four-wheel wagon can be helpful to pull supplies and plants, your garden journal and a plastic bottle of drinking water close to your garden.

❀ Keep tools and supplies where you can find them easily.

❀ Wear gardening gloves for weeding and trimming.

❀ Consider adding more plants, shrubs and trees you can hear. These might include the whispering of grasses, such as pampas grass (cortaderia selloana) and pearl grass (briza maxima) and the rustling of reeds and bamboo. Birch and pine trees create a soothing murmur as the wind tickles the branches.

❀ A water feature in the garden, such as a bubbling waterfall, helps orient a visually impaired gardener and creates a restful mood, too.

❀ Plant for texture and touch with plants that have soft, fuzzy leaves and flowers, like lamb's ear, pussy willow and Hare's Tale Grass (lagurus ovatus). Distinctive fragrances also can improve the garden by planting herbs such as basil and thyme, chamomile, lavender, lemon grass and lemon verbena.

❀ To make straight rows in vegetable gardens, tie knots in a rope as appropriate spacing for the mature plant, or have a helper do this for you. Then simply place a plant in at every knot.

❀ Using this knot system makes it easier to tell that the plants that do not line up with the knot are actually weeds.

❀ Consider using herbs and wild flowers to create a meadow effect in your garden. These do not require straight rows, but bring pleasure to the senses. Label or tag the plants to identify the varieties, in large print or in Braille. Even if you cannot see the lettering, a plant with a tag shouts, "Watch it, pal. I'm not a weed."

❀ Have a helper, if needed, describe a weed so that you can identify others. Smell the weed and feel the leaves and stem. To reduce the need to weed, use mulch between plants and rows. A layer of newspaper, while not attractive to the eye, works well as mulch and biodegrades during the growing season.

❀ Figuring out what's wrong with a plant and/or which diseases or bugs are bothering your blossoms is a chore for all gardeners. The visually impaired may need a helper to describe the ailment. While most gardeners prefer to use non-toxic sprays on plants and choose healthy, disease-resistant varieties to avoid dangerous chemicals, there may be times when you'll need the help of a sighted gardener to diagnosis and take care of sick plants.

For more information on gardening, you may want to consult with your local association for the blind.

The people-plant connection has been found, by horticultural therapists and we who sport green thumbs, to promote a heightened feeling of well being. Everyone, including the medical community, agrees working in the garden can relieve stress, increase relaxation, benefit social involvement, provide mental stimulation (including improved memory skills), improve balance and motor skills, enhance self-esteem and perhaps even heal the body.

There are recreational activities and socializing activities that special gardeners enjoy. In addition to the satisfaction, gardeners enjoy exercise and have improved mobility that includes the benefits of added muscle strength, flexibility and cardiopulmonary capability.

Those who garden in an enabled space need to work in the same dirt as everyone else in order to benefit from Nature's Health Plan. A number of companies have designed tools especially for the gardener with special needs, such as those that are lighter, designed for those with wrist or grip challenges and have longer padded foam handles. You can find them at garden centers or by searching the Internet. You can alter some of your own garden tools or become creative. For instance, you can plant peas without bending over by dropping the seed into the hole using a piece of plastic pipe.

According to author Lynn Dennis in *Garden for Life*, and other horticultural therapists, gardening has helped the physically disabled, the mentally ill, the developmentally disabled, the elderly, substance abusers, public offenders and the socially disadvantaged. The people in programs and at home connect with nature and the cycle of life. They can realize that they have an effect on something that is living, and often feel a reversal of dependence when they see how they function independently in the garden.

Age or experience level makes no difference in the can-do, enabled garden. People are too busy worrying about plants, vegetables, the soil and flowers, whether the weather is too hot or too cold, and how quickly seeds will sprout.

There is nothing pleasanter than spading
when the ground is soft and damp.
—John Steinbeck, author

Cultivate a Stronger Body:
The Shovel It Workout

Does the idea of gardening for fitness sound a whole lot more agreeable than dashing off to a crowded fitness center, lifting weights and jogging in circles around the track? Whether you're new to gardening or an old hand with a bright green thumb, the great news is that gardening is great exercise. It may take the place of other fitness routines or have a positive impact on your current workout.

Garden work, including mowing, shoveling, spading and weeding, can produce real and improved health benefits. According to the Mayo Clinic's health newsletter, "Hobbies do more than just pass the time…gardening and other diversions are tickets to better health. Gardening can condition the body, building strength, coordination and flexibility."

This fitness program, with the help of Nature, is good for your bones, which is smart news for all adults, especially women approaching, during and after menopausal years. Researchers at the University of Arkansas have linked regular yard work to the prevention of osteoporosis. It was found that women 50 and older who gardened at least once a week showed higher bone density readings (a very good thing, mind you) than those who performed other types of exercise. These other types included jogging, swimming, walking and even aerobic dance. The researchers didn't expect yard work to be significant. It's taken for such a dainty activity, many said. But as any gardener knows, there's a lot of weight-bearing motion going on in the garden, from digging holes and pulling weeds to hauling bags of humus and pushing a wheelbarrow.

An additional benefit of gardening is that it's an exercise that's performed outdoors. Exposure to sunlight boosts vitamin D production, which aids the body's ability to absorb calcium. That ability, along with the weight-bearing exercise, builds and strengthens bones. That means that Nature's giving you double your money's worth of rewards.

The best thing about gardening as a fitness routine is that most people are willing to do it. It doesn't inspire the same "Ack, not again!" feelings that other exercise programs often do.

Gardening is one place in life where we can workout alone, dressed in comfortable clothing, along with receiving the added benefit of reducing stress as we increase flexibility, burn calories and strengthen bones and muscles.

To be a fit gardener, take these tips to heart:

- ❀ Do several different types of activities in the garden. These might include turning the soil, raking leaves, digging holes for bulbs, planting vegetables, weeding. Plan to have each gardening workout last at least 5 minutes.
- ❀ So you don't experience that "I'm stiff all over" feeling at the end of the day or the next morning, switch positions and stance every few minutes. That is, crouch, then kneel, then stand, then bend. Stretch at the end of each workout.
- ❀ Exaggerate the motions you're doing while gardening, such as large sweeps when you get after the leaves with a rake.

❀ Stretch before extensive digging. Reach high over your head and try to touch the sky. Hold for a count of five, relax and repeat. Do some runner's lunges and rotate your shoulders. Never bob or bounce when stretching as this can damage muscles. After a gardening workout, stretch again. You might want to stretch before bed, too, especially if you haven't been in the garden for some time.

❀ Take extra care with your knees. Cover an old pillow or put one in a plastic trash bag on which to kneel as you garden. You may want to get a small stool with casters to roll around the garden. If the ground is rough, find a lightweight stool you can easily haul.

❀ Alternate your grip. If you're left handed, switch to your right hand while digging, and then switch back to your left hand.

❀ Give your back attention. Always lift with the thighs and keep your back straight. This sounds easy, but it's almost contrary to what a body wants to do when lifting a heavy object. Be careful not to twist as you lift, as this is often when back injuries occur. Invest in a lightweight wagon or dolly to haul bags of soil amendment into your garden. While hoeing, shoveling and raking, keep your knees relaxed.

❀ When bending forward from a standing position, such as when planting or trimming, bend from the hips, not the waist, which puts strain on the back.

❀ Never attempt to lift more than you can comfortably handle, and roll or push heavy loads.

❀ Wear gloves. I prefer the soft, but sturdy leather gloves that are made for women. They're a bit pricey, but I also like smooth hands. Yes, I've used the cotton ones and yes, they are machine washable, but for me they just don't last. Also, rose thorns are never thwarted by cotton gloves. Wear long sleeves if you're trimming prickly plants, such as berries, and consider the specially designed gloves that are leather up past the elbows. I like to apply a rich layer of hand cream before I put on my gloves so that my hands are getting moisturized as I work.

❀ Wear sturdy shoes or boots. It's tempting to wear the oldest sneakers on the planet for gardening, but remember, they weren't comfortable when you put them in the back of the closet and they won't be in the garden. Besides, you need foot protection out there.

❀ Select gardening tools and equipment that are comfortable for you to use. If you're using tools that are broken or rusty, you're probably not enjoying the garden as much as you could. Most women prefer short-handled shovels, taller women and men like the long-handled ones. Many companies are now producing tools for right and left handed gardeners and gardeners with disabilities or smaller hands.

❀ Wear a hat and sunscreen. Even on cloudy days the sun's rays can damage the skin.

❀ Give yourself a break. Do twenty minutes rather than a few hours. Sit in a comfortable spot, have a glass of water and enjoy the view.

❀ Gardening, like any fitness activity, requires us to replenish the water in our body. Drink plenty of water when in the garden. I like to take a few plastic bottles outside with me before I begin so that I don't have to take off muddy sneakers to dash inside. Thirst is an impulse we can overrule with our minds, and even a five percent loss of bodily fluid can make us feel out of sorts.

❀ For health reasons, always check with your physician before adding a new fitness routine to your schedule, especially if you have any concerns. And when talking with your doctor, find out if you're up to date on your tetanus shot. It makes good health sense, too, if you have any pain during gardening or have a wound that's not healing, to head for your doctor for assistance.

Studies show us that 30 minutes each day of moderate exercise, such as gardening, decreases the risk of numerous chronic ailments, including heart disease, stroke and Type-2 diabetes. According to sports medicine experts, gardening activities such as digging, raking and planting are the equivalent to sports such as snorkeling, volleyball and brisk walking. Tough gardening workouts, such as chopping wood, shoveling and tilling are on par with fencing, downhill skiing, softball and doubles tennis. In addition to gardening's physical benefits, the psychological boost conferred by accomplishing tasks can help shake off a feeling of helplessness.

Jeffrey P. Restuccio, author of *Fitness the Dynamic Gardening Way*, says, "Gardening is a Zen approach to health that gives you exercise, relief from stress, nutritious fruits and vegetables, companionship of family and friends and the aesthetic pleasures of working with nature. And it's an activity you can do all your life." Restuccio counsels, and Nature would agree, "Remember to enjoy the process, not just the product."

Think of gardening as an outdoor health spa and you'll increase your fitness level and have a luscious garden.

Here are some *Shovel It* fitness routines to get you started on Nature's ultimate exercise program. Start slowly with gardening as exercise, if you've been out of the yard for a while.

❀ Pick up that shovel, business end over your right shoulder, and hold it high over your head. Keep arms straight, shoulders relaxed and hips forward. Bend your knees slightly. Now slowly turn at the waist. This is a weight lifting and stretching exercise, so it's to be done at a snail's pace. Need to see snails in action? Just come to my garden. Now relax and switch sides, that is, have the actual shovel part of the tool over your left shoulder.

❀ Push a long-handled shovel into the earth and hold it with one hand for balance. Stand with feet slightly apart and tighten the muscles throughout the calves, thighs and buttocks as you go up on your toes. Go up and down for a count of 20. This will help condition your largest muscle groups. Remember to breathe deeply as you work out. Relax and do another set of 20.

❀ To strengthen the abdominal area, which in turn supports the muscles in a healthy, strong and pain-free back, do this exercise every chance you get. Simply contract your stomach muscles for a slow count of five. Relax and repeat five more times. Warning: This exercise is addictive and you may find that you're doing it while weeding, hoeing and even driving your car or sitting at the computer. No problem, however, because it's good for you and can help flatten your tummy.

❀ To strength the upper torso and increase flexibility, simply push shoulders forward and hold for a count of five. Relax and then push shoulders back, arching your spine slightly. Now relax again and lift your chin to the sky, hold and relax.

Kids, seniors and others in your life can garden right along with you, for the health of it, but you have to be the working example.

If you're planting a fitness seed with your gardening, you may want to incorporate other exercise programs into your life, including yoga and walking.

Earth laughs in flowers.
—Ralph Waldo Emerson

*One of the most endearing qualities
of gardeners, though it makes their gardens
worse, is this faculty of being
too easily delighted.
—Henry Mitchell, master gardener,
journalist, author*

Say Ah: Yoga, Relaxation for the Gardening Soul

"Way, way back then," as a senior friend likes to say when referring to things of the past, yoga was performed by gurus and health nuts. Things change, thank heavens, and now all age groups practice yoga. It's popular with Gen-Xers as well as Baby Boomers who want a good stretch and a sound workout. Yoga improves concentration, promotes well being and helps the body's ability to stay flexible. Along with gardening, it could be physical insurance for later in life.

Now that I've given you a "teaser" about later in life, let me introduce a thought that could save your bones when you're in your sixties, seventies, eighties and beyond. As we age, we often lose strength and bone density. New medications may change that and a determination to stay strong may keep us more powerful, but we still need a good sense of balance. Recently I discovered that those who practice yoga and practice balancing are less likely to trip and tumble later in life. To me that's reason enough to participate in this program, and if you can perform yoga outdoors in the sunlight or shade you'll get an added bonus of being exposed to natural Vitamin D, which helps the body absorb calcium. Why not add a spot for a yoga workout when working on your Garden Bubble or when you physically make changes in your garden.

Here is some yoga information, and as you read, I urge you to find a class and try it for just six weeks. Most community colleges and community recreation departments have classes. You can find videos that will take you through the movements, and there are books on the topic, too.

There are different types of yoga.

Ashtanga is sometimes called Power Yoga. In this form, you'll be jumping from one posture to the next, working up a sweat and getting a great physical workout. You'll move quickly through the routines.

Dhyann is meditation that occurs during a yoga session.

Iyengar promotes body alignment. You'll spend time focusing on your body's position and control.

Kundalini focuses on how breath moves through the body, especially up and down the spine. This form of yoga may include meditation and chanting. Many devotees believe that Kundalini is the most relaxing type of yoga.

Take a beginner's class if you're new to yoga. You will be asked to try the positions as the instructor explains how to do each correctly. Listen carefully and ask questions. Sports injuries can occur in a yoga class when participants do not stretch or move properly.

Try the different styles of yoga. If you've been doing heavy gardening chores, such as chopping wood, hauling amendments and shoveling compost, Ashtanga yoga might be a good cross-training workout and still give you an energized program. Likewise, Iyengar yoga may prove to be the stress relieving routine that balances a more vigorous fitness program. Kundalini yoga may just make you feel wonderful.

Here are some yoga words you'll want to know as you begin:

Asanas: exercise postures or positions

Dhyann: meditation

Mantra: meditative sound, prayers

Pranayama: deep breathing

Yogi: yoga teacher

Yogin: male yoga teacher

Yogini: female yoga teacher

Here's a yoga posture that's simple and refreshing. Why not try it right now?

Take off your shoes so that your toes can slightly grip the grass of your lawn or an outdoor carpet. You'll want to be on a soft surface, rather than a concrete patio. You may put your free hand on your hip or place it in the middle of your chest.

Now holding the edge of a sturdy chair or the railing of the deck, comfortably place your right foot on the floor. Take a slow breath and put your left foot on the inside of your right calf. If you're comfortable and feel safe, raise your left foot to the side of your knee or the middle of your thigh.

Balance in this position for a count of ten. If you're comfortable, continue for a count of 50. Slowly allow your left foot to return to the floor and repeat on the opposite side.

Remember, you want to relax, concentrate on your body and forget the burdens of your mind. Breathe slowly.

In a yoga class, you might also do a posture like this. Your ultimate goal is to balance without the aid of a chair or wall and with only one foot on the floor as you relax.

Yoga makes sense to me. Try it and see how good you can feel.

*The main purpose of a garden
is to give its owner the best and highest kind
of earthly pleasure.
—Gertrude Jekyll, gardener, author*

J Meditate, Therefore J Am

To enhance your workout, it's time to learn to relax. Yes, a day in the vegetable garden will do that, but what happens if you come home late? It's already dark, but still nice outdoors and you need to unwind. Here's a five-step gardener's meditation to do anytime.

In order to release stress and enjoy the meditation, you'll want to select a place where you can be comfortable and alone. I hope you've designated an area in your garden for meditation. Remember, it need not be fancy. In my garden there's a huge stump where I can sit, enjoy a bit of sun and relax. It's quiet, I cannot see any neighbors' homes and there's lots of greenery around.

You may want to sit at the park, in a public garden, your house of worship's prayer garden or even an open field. You may want to arrange some plants around you as you meditate. Choose a location where you are safe, since you'll be relaxed and need to close your eyes.

Thoughts do affect wellness. If you're constantly berating yourself, from having a black thumb to being too critical about any of your physical or intellectual parts, that's what your mind believes. This also applies if there are people in your life who are critical, hurtful and all-out objectionable. You may frequently hear that faultfinding voice.

Instead, meditate on your positive qualities and you'll help yourself to achieve better feelings about your life and even your garden. Do you recall the "green thumb effect" we discussed previously? That same theory can affect how you're nurturing your mind and your body.

Now sit in a relaxed position or lie on a padded surface. Close your eyes. You may want to recite the following onto a tape recorder so that you don't have to memorize it or open your eyes after you begin. It's easy and can be helpful for the entire family.

Withdraw. Pull away from everything around you. Don't reject your life or resist problems, simply turn your attention inward. Take a mini vacation from strife. Think of a turtle and how she pulls her head and legs into the shell.

Affirm. Give yourself some positive feedback and project positive images about yourself. You might try repeating, "Nature is blessing me." "I am at peace." "I am strong and healthy."

Create. Project your thoughts to a point in the middle of your forehead and think of this as the sun in the universe. Feel all your troubles go to that one point.

Focus. Strive to feel peace and goodness flow from your "sun point" out through your body. You'll feel your body becoming lighter.

Look forward. Breathe deeply and allow the fresh air of your garden to cleanse your blood, your bones and your brain. Allow feelings of well being to flow back with each inhalation.

Don't think. Push away all thoughts and just be. When you're ready, stretch and slowly return to reality.

A variation of this meditation can be done anywhere you can relax and be safe, such as in your garden.

Sitting comfortably or lying on a padded surface, fix your gaze on a flower, a plump vegetable, a slice of fruit or any plant. Say the name of this part of nature over and over, clearing out other thoughts that have muddied your day. For instance, I might say, "Rose, rose, rose, rose…" Or, call it by its name: "Vanilla Perfume, Vanilla Perfume, Vanilla Perfume…"

At this time study the flower or plant. Look at the leaves, the coloration, the petals, the texture and the stems.

When you're ready, stop saying the plant's name and just begin to examine it. Allow your mind to only concentrate on this object. Try sitting for about 10 minutes. Some people who meditate do it for 30 minutes to an hour a day, and that's fine if you have time. I never do.

After you feel more relaxed or your mind is at rest, begin to contract and then release the muscles in your body. Start with your toes and move to your face and finally the top of your head. You may want to sit a bit longer and ponder life, but whatever you do, get up slowly. Pretend you're a wet dog and shake your body. Exhale and inhale deeply. Straighten your posture and you'll feel more ready to tackle whatever life has in store.

Meditation has been proven to lower blood pressure and promote feelings of wellness. Many find that taking a meditation class helps; others can easily pick up the method, or a method that agrees with one's needs. Meditation is grounded in Christianity, as well as Asian religions, and it basically allows the mind to settle down. A relaxed mind and body can promote healing and speed recovery after illness. As such, you may find that after a meditation session, you're more clearly focused on what is in your heart, more so than ever before.

Prayer is conversation with God.
—Clement of Alexandria

As I draw near the borderland...
the wonderful light of the other life seems
often to shine so joyfully into this one,
that I almost forget the past and present,
in an eager anticipation
of the approaching awakening.
—Elizabeth Blackwell, M.D.,
Pioneer Work for Women
(first woman physician in the United States)

This Breath's for Me

The garden, whether it's your balcony, a public park or straight out your living room door, is the right place to practice breathing. Yes, yes, of course. I know you've been doing it since birth. But let's be real, we typically don't get sufficient oxygen. If you've been sitting at a computer, behind the steering wheel of your car or deeply involved in a knotty problem, you're probably not getting enough air. The results may range from a headache to depression to a mild feeling of resentment.

What can better breathing do for you? In addition to a good way to relax, better breathing and deep breathing can reduce discomforts and fear of pain, including chronic pain, reduce nervousness for new non-smokers, and restore well being for those with headache, low-back pain, joint pain. Deep breathing has been shown to relax those undergoing chemotherapy and victims of cancer and AIDS. According to the Internet source MedLine (July 31, 1999), if you're not breathing well, you may be suffering needlessly.

Here's a variation on a deep-breathing technique based on some of the ideas offered by psychiatrist Karen Syrjala and *The Management of Cancer Pain.*

You'll want to sit in a quiet place where you won't be interrupted. Think about something that makes you happy or feel good. If you're unable to be in a garden, set your mind's eye to your own garden, your heart's garden or a real garden you've visited. Concentrate on this image. To relax your facial muscles, which can aid in the positive effects of deep breathing. You may want to screw up your face, much like we all did as children when something tasted really terrible. Hold that look for a moment and then relax.

With your mouth closed and your shoulders relaxed, inhale through your nose slowly and deeply. You'll do this to a slow count of four. Try to fill your lungs from the lowest part to the highest part, pushing out your abdomen, then your lower ribs, then your chest as your body fills with air. Hold your breath for a count of three or four. Now through your mouth, exhale as you let out as much air as possible, starting with the lowest point of your lungs and moving to the highest.

Repeat for five to ten minutes. If you become lightheaded, alternate six normal breaths with six deep breaths.

In *HealthCentral's* "What Can People Do on Their Own to Relieve Chronic Pain?" Dr. Bart Goldman says that to stay healthy and help heal the body, one must breath deeply and take at least 10 to 20 minutes a day, just for yourself, whether it's meditation or prayer, stress management or for deep breathing. "I've never had a patient not improve if they have taken this advice."

Chapter 6

Asleep in the Moonlight

*If we persist, I do not doubt that by age 96
or so we will all have gardens we are
pleased with, more or less.*
—Henry Mitchell,
master gardener and author

Just ask 'em: Why do you garden? The garden-variety gardener will say simple things, "I love the fresh vegetables and fruits." Another will respond, "I like the outdoors." And about one in every ten gardeners will say, "The smell." If you've ever deeply breathed in the lusty, addictive perfume of soil, the odor that comes about after turning a shovel filled with black earth, you know of what they speak.

It's better than any fragrance put out by any perfume company. It produces stuff guaranteed to snag you your soul and have you cup a handful of soil. It's fresh, sweet and addictive. So rather than ask another gardener or yourself what you like best about Nature's Health Plan, describe the effect on your senses when you inhale moist soil, crushed herbs, violets, lilacs and moist leaves on an October afternoon just when the sunshine is fading.

In this chapter we're going to talk about the aromas of the garden, beginning with the language of flowers and how you might want to design a secret into your garden, one that could become a lusty love letter, if you so desire. Here we'll stroll through the garden and discover what trees can tell about you. Yes, they have some secrets up their branches, and if you're creating a garden, you might want to include your tree. This chapter reveals ways to capture the aroma of the garden and produce exotic effects, perhaps even enchanting Ms. or Mr. Right in the process. Aroma experts suggest that if you place a piece of orange peel in your pocket, people will be drawn to you, people like potential partners for romance. In addition to aromatherapy, we'll talk about herbs and why life could feel much better if you plant just a few in that window box or backyard.

So, settle your chair in the sunshine or next to the fire, and begin to breathe in the essence of aromatherapy that's much a part of Nature's Health Plan. Why not sleep in the moonlight tonight, or just hang out in the garden as the stars come into view. The garden can become a whole new wonderful world when cloaked in darkness.

Flowers are the sweetest things
God ever made and forgot
to put a soul into.
—Reverend Henry Ward Beecher,
author, advocate and father
of Harriet Beecher Stow

> No poet I've ever heard of has written an
> ode to a load of manure. Somebody should,
> and I'm not trying to be funny.
> —Ruth Stout, gardener and author

What Flowers Really Say

There's a language in flowers. If you could ask any Victorian lady or gentlemen, you'd surely get an earful of advice. What? You didn't study this language in any school or college class? My goodness, and you thought you were well educated. Well, you are in luck. Here are the meanings of flowers so that the next time you give a bouquet, you can pass along a secret.

Once you acquire the code for the language of flowers, why, you might want to plant buttercups, dianthus and baby's breath in a planter and tell those in the know that, "I'll never forget you." You could give a bouquet of ivy and fern to your love and say, "Your fidelity is fascinating." Throw in a bunch of white clover to this arrangement and make the plea, "Think of me." Add some verbena and your message states, "Pray for me."

Woe to the one who receives a bouquet of lettuce (cold heartedness), peony (shame), primrose (I can't live without you) and a mock orange (deceit). We're talking dangerous liaisons here and buckets of issues. It doesn't take the brains of a linguist or a rocket scientist, once you understand the code, to see that something is amiss and the receiver should watch out.

Speaking with flowers, though wildly popular in Britain and America during the Victorian era, the language began in the 1600s in Constantinople (now Istanbul), Turkey. According to floral history, the language and art of flowers was introduced to England by Lady Mary Wortley in 1716, after she returned from living in Turkey with her husband. Everyone who was anyone jumped on the flower-language bandwagon, and in no time at all, the French were taking it to new heights. The first book of the language, *Book Le Language des Fleurs*, suggested more than 800 floral combinations. Floral historians say that when the book was translated to English, the meanings of the combinations had to be toned down because most were risqué and would have horrified Her Majesty, Queen Victoria.

How can designing with the language of flowers make you happier, healthier and more peaceful? Simple. It returns a sense of play, relaxation and whimsy to life. We need more play, and yet as supposedly adult humans, we're often not allowed that life-giving opportunity. Find your playful soul in flowers. You'll find some reference guides on flower speak in the library or bookstore if you want to delve into this language further. As you plant your garden, consider secretly spelling out "Love Is Eternal" or writing about trust, fidelity and cheerfulness with your plant and flower choices.

Amaryllis: Pastoral poetry

Apple blossom: Preference

Aster: Symbol of love

Azalea: Take care of yourself, fragile, passion, womanhood

Baby's breath: Pure of heart

Bachelor's button: Single blessedness

Begonia: Beware

Bluebell: Humility

Buttercup: Riches

Cactus: Endurance

Camellia: Admiration, perfection, gratitude, longing for you

Cape jasmine: Secret love

Cattail: Peace, prosperity

Chrysanthemum: You're a wonderful friend, truth, cheerfulness

Crocus: Cheerfulness, gladness

Daffodil: Unrequited love, respect, regard

Dahlia: Dignity, elegance

Daisy: Innocence, loyal love, purity

Fern: Magic, grace, fascination, secret bond of love

Fir: Time

Forsythia: Anticipation

Foxglove: Insincerity

Freesia: Trust

Garlic: Courage, strength

Geranium: Stupidity, folly

Gladiola: Trust, I'm sincere

Gloxinia: Love at first sight

Goldenrod: Success

Holly: Am I forgotten?

Honeysuckle: Devoted love, fidelity

Hydrangea: Thank you for understanding

Iris: Faith, hope, wisdom, valor, my compliments

Jasmine: Grace and elegance

Larkspur: Fickleness

Lavender: Admiration, solitude, protection, wishes come true

Lily: Beauty, youth, gratitude

Lily of the Valley: Sweetness, humility, you've made my life

Mistletoe: Kiss me, affection

Oleander: Caution

Orange blossoms: Eternal love, marriage, fruitful

Orange, Mock: Deceit

Orchid: Mature charm

Pansy: Merriment

Peony: Shame, compassion

Petunia: Resentment, anger, your presence soothes me

Pine: Hope, pity

Poppy: Pleasure, consolation, imagination

Primrose: I can't live without you

Rose: Love (and more)

Snapdragon: Deception, strength

Stock: Bonds of affection, promptness

Sunflower: Pride

Sweet William: Gallantry

Sweet pea: Goodbye, pleasure, thank you for a lovely time

Tulip: Perfect lover, luck

Violet: Modesty, virtue, faithfulness

Wild rose: Simplicity

Wisteria: Welcome

Zinnia: I mourn your absence, daily remembrance

Carnations have a language of their own. Carnations express love, fascination and distinction. Purple carnations indicate capriciousness; pink have the greatest historical significance. According to a Christian legend, carnations first appeared as Jesus carried the Cross. Shedding tears as she helplessly watched the procession, carnations sprang up wherever the Virgin Mary's tears fell to the earth. The pink carnation has become the symbol of a mother's undying love. In 1907, the pink carnation was chosen as the emblem for Mother's Day.

Rose colors have spectacular meanings. Red roses of any shade mean, "I love you." White roses signify spiritual love and purity. Pink roses, such as those in a bridal bouquet mean, "Happy love." Yellow roses mean joy and gladness, but in Victorian times meant a decrease of love and infidelity. Coral-colored roses signify desire. Orange says, "I'm fascinated and enthusiastic about you." Lavender roses mean, "It's love at first sight." Light pink roses mean grace, gentility and admiration, while dark pink roses say, "Thank you." All pale shades of roses allow you to say, "Thank you and you're my friend" in the language of flowers.

The grouping of roses speaks volumes to a lover's heart. Two roses joined together means an engagement. One deep red rose means bashful shame and a bunch of red and white roses together signifies unity. And if you blend moss, rose and myrtle, you've just confessed your adoration. A dozen roses is the ultimate declaration of love and devotion. Red and yellow roses in a bouquet tell the receiver, "I'm happy for you." And to communicate your passionate nature, just give someone a bouquet of yellow and orange roses. But should one receive a rose devoid of thorns and leaves, the message is clear: "There's no hope for us."

So the next time you simply pick a bouquet to give to a co-worker, friend or lover, you'd better watch what you're saying, especially now that you speak flower-ese.

It is in winter that trees reveal what they
most truly are—alien presences possessed
of a stark and foreign beauty that owes little
to the human race.
—Allen Lacy, author and gardener

A Tree By Another Name

Would you like to increase your prosperity? Then you might want to plant a cedar tree in your garden. Want to have your life become more fertile? Then according to ancient lore, you should plant a fig tree.

In many cultures and traditions, the plants that surround us have specific symbolism. Using Celtic lore, for example, trees have spirits and energies. As you personalize your garden, you may want to include this mythology in your plans. Just as flowers have meaning, so do trees. The tree is the primary Celtic symbol. It is believed that the tree is a bridge between the land and sky, heaven and earth. In the lore, trees communicate through water between these realms and all realms are united within the tree.

If you'd like to follow these practices, you may want to plant according to the mythology of the ancient Celts who lived in Scotland, Ireland, England and much of Europe eons ago.

Almond: Divination, clairvoyance, wisdom, money and business

Alder: Protection against oracular powers

Apple: Associated with healing, prosperity, love and perpetual youth, innocence. It represents choice.

Apricot: Connected with love and beauty

Ash: Links the inner and outer worlds and is used in purification, including mental purification. Recommended for protection, as well as protection on the seas and against sea magic.

Beech: Associated with stability and flow of energy

Birch: Symbolizes rebirth, purification and new beginnings

Blackthorn: Represents unexpected change and a radical rebirth after a stormy conception

Cedar: Thought to increase prosperity and longevity and repel negative energies

Cypress: Thought to be a tree of remembrance and mourning

Dogwood: Believed to add charm and social standing

Elder: Represents the end in the beginning and the beginning in the end

Elm: Used as protection against evil areas and to ward off wrong-doers

Fig: Considered the symbol of fertility, strength, energy and health

Fir: Symbolizes malleability, cleverness and ability to change

Hawthorn: Believed to be a symbol to ward off strife and harshness. Planted as a protection to dispel negative energies.

Hazel: Represents marriage and protection

Hazelnut: Symbolizes attraction, loss of inhibition or will power or drowsiness

Heather: Considered to help people feel stable and grounded, with the ability to listen to what their bodies are saying

Hemlock: Thought to be negative in Celtic lore, and gardeners were admonished not to use it.

Holly: Symbolizes life with its challenges, the need to achieve unity and many working together to achieve goals

Lemon: Considered to improve abilities of divination and healing

Lime: Represents chastity and neutrality

Juniper: Planted around homes for protection

Maple: Believed to increase powers of divination and love. The tree supposedly increases cohesiveness.

Mulberry: Thought to increase knowledge, wisdom and self-will

Oak: Used widely in ancient Celtic lore. Symbolizes healing strength, money, power, authority, majesty and all that is good

Olive: Symbolizes peace, fruitfulness, security and money

Orange: Believed to increase love and marriage

Pine: Represents purification, good health, abundance, fertility and prosperity

Reed: Symbolizes music

Rowan: Thought to increase strength and protection against negative or enchanting charms

Sequoia: Used to increase longevity and promote wisdom

Sycamore: Considered to enhance spiritual growth

Walnut: Used for healing and protection

White poplar: Believed to help overcome hurdles

Willow: Symbolizes protection from enchantment and used for the speedy and easy delivery of babies

Yew: Represents transformation and rebirth

Like the signs of the zodiac, each of us is supposed to have a "tree" of our birth, which some believe describes our personalities. Just for fun, you might want to plant your Birth Tree according to the following information. Just find your birthday, note your tree and then refer to the description that follows.

January 1 to January 11 - Fir tree

January 12 to January 24 - Elm tree

January 25 to February 3 – Cypress tree

February 4 to February 8 - Poplar tree

February 9 to February 18 - Cedar tree

February 19 to Feb 29 - Pine tree

March 1 to March 10 - Weeping Willow tree

March 11 to March 20 - Lime tree

March 21 - Oak tree

March 22 to March 31 - Hazelnut tree

April 1 to Apr 10 - Rowan tree

April 11 to April 20 - Maple tree

April 21 to April 30 - Walnut tree

May 1 to May 14 - Poplar tree

May 15 to May 24 - Chestnut tree

May 25 to June 3 - Ash tree

June 4 to June 13 - Hornbeam tree

June 14 to June 23 - Fig tree

June 24 – Birch tree

June 25 to July 4 - Apple tree

July 5 to July 14 – Fir tree

July 15 to July 25 - Elm tree

July 26 to August 4 - Cypress tree

August 5 to August 13 - Poplar tree

August 14 to August 23 - Cedar tree

August 24 to September 2 - Pine tree

September 3 to September 12 - Weeping Willow tree

September 13 to September 22 - Lime tree

September 23 - Olive tree

September 24 to October 3 - Hazelnut tree

October 4 to October 13 - Rowan tree

October 14 to October 23 - Maple tree

October 24 to November 11 - Walnut tree

November 12 to November 21 - Chestnut tree

November 22 to December 1 - Ash tree

December 2 to December 11 - Hornbeam tree

December 12 to December 21 - Fig tree

December 22 - Beech tree

December 23 to December 31 - Apple tree

APPLE TREE: Those born to the apple tree have oodles of charm, flair and sex appeal. This person easily attracts others and always has a pleasant aura about him or her. The apple tree denotes a flirtatious, adventurous, sensitive nature, one who is always in love, wants to love and be loved. This person may be in love with life, too. The apple tree is a faithful and tender partner and is generous. He or she has a logical mind, scientific talents, lives for today yet brims with zest for tomorrow, and has the persona of a carefree philosopher with imagination.

ASH TREE: Those who are born to the ash tree are uncommonly attractive, vivacious, impulsive and demanding. He or she does not care for criticism and can be easily offended. The ash tree is ambitious, intelligent and talented but likes to play with fate. There may be an egotistic personality side, but the ash tree is reliable and trustworthy. You won't find a more faithful and prudent lover, yet sometimes the brain rules over the heart, both in business and pleasure, and then relationships become rocky. The ash tree takes all partnerships seriously.

BEECH TREE: Those who are born to the beech tree have good taste, whether that concerns outward appearance or a sense of style. He or she may be materialistic, yet seem blasé about money. The beech tree is a good organizer in life and career, with a logical and economical mannerism. The beech tree makes an excellent leader, takes no unnecessary risks, is reasonable and is a splendid lifetime companion in love or business.

BIRCH TREE: Those who are born to the birch tree are vivacious, attractive, elegant, friendly, unpretentious and yet modest. He or she does not like anything in excess, abhors the vulgar, loves life in nature. You'll see the birch tree dressed in cotton and earth tones, and there's an aura of calm surrounding this person. However, he or she is full of imagination, has less ambition, and will attempt in any relationship to create a contented environment.

CEDAR TREE: Those who are born to the cedar tree are of rare beauty. These are the people who walk into a room and are noticed in seconds. The cedar tree doesn't just like luxury, he or she must have it, even if it's in very small, but precious things. He or she is not the least shy and is self-confident, determined and impatient. There's a tendency with the cedar tree to try to impress others, and often does because this person has many talents, is industrious, has a healthy optimism and is able to make quick, correct decisions. While the cedar may have flirtations, he or she may wait years for one true love.

CHESTNUT TREE: Those who are born to the chestnut tree ooze elegance and strength. They have a well-developed sense of justice and avoid boasting. Most are vivacious, interested in others more than themselves and are born to be a diplomat, but irritate easily. The chestnut tree may be sensitive and quiet in a crowd, which seems to go against their outward appearance, but at times they lack confidence.

As a result, it may seem like he or she is trying to be aloof and superior. The chestnut tree may only love deeply once in a lifetime and often feels that he or she will never find the right partner.

CYPRESS TREE: Those born to the cypress tree are strong, faithful, muscular and compliant. This person can take what life gives out with a smile, and can muster determination regardless of the crisis. He or she is content, optimistic and fun to be around. The cypress tree craves money and acknowledgment. He or she enjoys being alone, but hates to be lonely. The cypress tree is a gentle, passionate lover, who is satisfied with a faithful partner. There's also a quick-tempered and unruly side to the cypress tree.

ELM TREE: Those born to the elm tree are attractive, and while they might say they're just average, others would like to have their handsomeness. The elm tree has excellent taste, especially in clothing, rarely demands and is cheerful. He or she, however, tends to remember the mistakes of others. The elm tree likes to lead and has the ability to see the big picture with a strong practical side. The elm tree is honest, makes a faithful partner, is generous and has a wonderful sense of humor.

FIG TREE: Those born to the fig tree have strong personalities and may be accused of being too independent and self-willed. He or she doesn't allow arguments or challenges to stop progress, whether in love or life. Family, children and animal companions are an important part of the fig tree's life. He or she is a bit of a social butterfly, has a well-grounded sense of humor and enjoys being lazy. The fig tree is talented, practical and typically has an above-average intelligence level.

FIR TREE: Those born to the fir tree have extraordinary taste, which may range from selecting friends to drinking tea to only eating the finest chocolates or caviar. He or she is dignified, sophisticated, and loves anything beautiful. The fir tree tends to be moody, stubborn and quiet at times. He or she may be modest yet ambitious, talented and determined. The fir tree is a faithful lover, has many friends, few foes and rarely says one thing and does another. Need advice? Come to the fir tree. You can depend on the fir tree.

HAZELNUT TREE: Those born to the hazelnut tree are charming, undemanding, understanding and lovingly know how to make a good impression. The hazelnut tree is typically an activist or promotes various social causes. This person is popular, honest, tolerant, precise and has a good value system. The hazelnut may be a capricious lover, but knows the merit of a faithful relationship.

HORNBEAM TREE: Those born to the hornbeam tree have a cool beauty about them. He or she has exquisite taste, and while often wealthy, there's nothing egotistical about the hornbeam tree. He or she wants to make life comfortable and figures out how to do it. This person leads a disciplined life and looks for the kindness in others, so when seeking a romantic partner, the hornbeam tree is often cautious before making a commitment.

LIME TREE: Those born to the lime tree accept whatever life serves up and does it with style and composure. He or she hates arguments (although will argue if necessary), dislikes laziness and prizes hard work. The lime tree will make huge sacrifices for friends and family, including romantic partners, but he or she is not foolish in love. The lime tree is creative, multitalented, is tenacious and works without complaining. There's a jealous side to the lime tree that few but an inner circle of loyal friends ever see.

MAPLE TREE: Those born to the maple tree have higher-than-average intelligence. Here is someone filled with imagination, ambition, pride and self-confidence and who is smart, even if she or he lacks "school learning." The maple tree strives to impress others, hungers for new experiences, may be fidgety, can have many sides to a personality and often has a complicated love life. The maple tree has a good memory, which comes in handy when love is complicated.

OAK TREE: Those who are born to the oak tree are brave, whether that's in the workaday world or in the midst of a family crisis. The oak tree has excellent health and a robust nature. He or she is strong physically and strong-willed, too. The oak tree is independent, sensible, sometimes inflexible and often detests change. The oak tree is a person of action who keeps an eye on the big picture of life.

OLIVE TREE: Those born to the olive tree are filled with wisdom. If you need a shoulder to cry on or someone to help decide if you should change careers, it's probably an olive tree you should call. The olive tree loves the sun and outdoors life. He or she is warm-hearted and friendly, always saying just the right kind words to others. This person seeks a practical love partner, but one with a sophisticated side, and will go to almost any length to avoid aggressive people or behavior. The olive tree is tolerant, with a sense of justice.

PINE TREE: Those born to the pine tree love to find joyful company and seek out friends who are also upbeat and positive. The pine tree is healthy and robust and strives to make life comfortable. He or she is very active and a comfortable and natural companion. The pine tree falls in love easily, but the passion may quickly burn out until the right person comes along. This may lead to disappointments in the life of the practical, trustworthy pine tree.

POPLAR TREE: Those born to the poplar tree are often brave on the outside, but quaking internally. He or she is attractive and knows how to play up those natural good looks. The poplar tree needs to live in beautiful surroundings, is choosy with jobs and friends and has a strong artistic nature. The poplar tree is a great organizer and will lead with a firm and practical manner. He or she is reliable and takes all partnerships, including those of the heart, seriously.

ROWAN TREE: Those born to the rowan tree are sensitive and full of charm. He or she is upbeat and cheerful, with little egotism involved. The rowan tree does, however, like to draw attention, whether at work or in love. Life is always in motion for the rowan tree, and he or she can be both independent and dependent. There's a strong artistic side to the rowan tree's nature, which makes for an emotional roller coaster, especially since there's a tendency to forget that others are human.

WALNUT TREE: Those born to the walnut tree are passionate by nature, whether in love or working for a cause. He or she can be so focused that trivial things like buying birthday presents for a loved one are forgotten. The walnut tree has a noble, regal bearing, loves the unexpected and may be inflexible and even aggressive at times. Compromise isn't a concept easily understood by this person. The walnut tree may not always be liked, but he or she is always admired.

WEEPING WILLOW: Those born to the weeping willow have a thoughtful, perhaps melancholy side. This individual loves beauty, is often extremely attractive and has incredible taste. The weeping willow is empathetic, a dreamer, honest and influential. Since he or she can be demanding at times, love affairs often start on unsteady ground, but the weeping willow has a knack for reading people intuitively. The weeping willow may suffer in relationships, yet when a steady, kind lover or partner comes along, there's a perfect match.

A solitary maple on a woodside flames in single scarlet, recalls nothing so much as the daughter of a noble house dressed for a fancy ball, with the whole family gathered round to admire her before she goes.
—Henry James, author

*I believe a leaf of grass is no less than the
journey-work of the stars.*
—Walt Whitman, American Poet

Smell Power

Aromatherapy is a big word that simply means, "This smells good." Typically the person doing the smelling takes a second breath because the first was so pleasurable. The use of natural plant perfumes and oils is much discussed these days, especially as many people routinely consult complementary or alternative health methods along with traditional medical practices.

Technically, aromatherapy is the inhalation and bodily application of essential oils from aromatic plants in order to relax, balance, rejuvenate, restore or enhance body, mind and spirit. Pure essential oils, used in aromatherapy, are extracted from plant parts such as the flower, leaf, bark, root, twig, seed, berry, rind, resin and bulb. The basic principle of aromatherapy is to strengthen the self-healing processes by indirect stimulation of the immune system.

Because it's not possible, without extensive funding, to do blind studies and devote years of research on the use of common plants and flowers to make you feel better, there's little scientific data to support aromatherapy. But really now, if inhaling in the fragrance of a rose helps you forget your troubles for even a second, I believe it's cause for applause. That's nature at work, and you just have to breathe.

Here's the scoop on aromatherapy. The results of using essential oils, plants and flowers as part of Nature's Health Plan are individual. Aromatherapy textbooks and websites recommend uses for specific oils and plants, as no two people will be affected the same way. Further, depending on the situation, mood or time of day or month, an aromatherapy may have a totally opposite result than it had previously.

The history of aromatherapy pre-dates written records. Combinations of oils, resins and fragrant plants have been used in religious, ceremonial and mystical celebrations and in spells and cures in even the most ancient of civilizations. Some of the earliest documented uses come from ancient Egypt where 3,000-or-more-year-old papyruses show that aromatherapy was used to cure illnesses, as skin care products, massage oils and cosmetics, and to maintain the bodies of those heading for the afterlife.

The Chinese Yellow Emperor Book of Internal Medicine, written about 2697 BC, is the oldest surviving medical book in China and contains listings of more than 300 plants and their medicinal qualities. Aromatherapies were used in Greece and Rome. The Romans were so enamored with scented oils that they extended trade routes to East India, Arabia and beyond to secure the precious substances. Ayurveda, traditional Indian medicine, has been practiced for more than 3,000 years, and massages using fragrant oils have always been a key part of it. The Aztecs, Incas and Mayans used aromatic plants and oils in rituals and daily life. North American native peoples used aromatic oils, plants and plant extracts in rites, ceremonies, celebrations and medicine.

The term "aromatherapy" was coined in 1928 by the French chemist Rene-Maurice Gattefosse, and the good doctor probably would never have imagined that today aromatherapy is a $300 million business and growing. In Europe it is often considered an essential part of one's health program, and insurance companies commonly pay for treatments. In the United States aromatherapy is still considered alternative or complementary therapy.

Essential oils are highly distilled substances produced for the oils you can buy at the store. Most would be toxic if swallowed, so it's mandatory to keep everything out of the reach of children, pets or adults for whom safety is mandatory.

Those who embrace and practice aromatherapy give warnings: The oils are highly concentrated and, until diluted with other oils or non-fragrant creams or alcohol, may burn the skin. For instance, if one is using an essential oil in an inhalant, just adding five to ten drops of oil to steaming water would be plenty.

Essential oils can be used as massage oils when diluted with a light oil, referred to as carrier oil, such as sweet almond. Contrary to urban myths, essential oils (and actually any oils at all) cannot penetrate the skin and be absorbed into the bloodstream. The skin is the largest organ of the body and is designed to keep contaminants out. Medical patches are designed to deliver medication through the skin; essential oils do not penetrate the skin. The oils used in massage are breathed through the nose and therefore provide a feeling of tranquillity and the possible healthful effects of the fragrance.

Aromatherapy can be included in baths with a small amount of the fragrant oil placed in hot water. You can also add flowers and herbs wrapped in a measure of cheesecloth to the bath for a relaxing soak, too.

For a stuffy head, try an inhalation of fragrant oils or plants and leaves. I like to infuse (it's like making a strong tea) peppermint leaves for an inhalation when my head feels congested. Essential oils and fragrant plants and flowers will burn your eyes, so keep them closed. I like to use an infusion of cinnamon stick in water and then spritz it around the house. You may want to add one or two drops of orange oil to a spray bottle and spritz clothing before adding the laundry to the dryer.

You can create your own perfume by adding 25 drops of an essential oil that pleases your nose to 1 ounce of water or an oil, such as grape seed or sweet almond oil. Keep the mixture in a mist spray bottle.

Here are some other uses for oils that are available online, at bath and body lotion stores and at cosmetic shops. The plants and flowers can also come from your garden, but they will not be as potent. Yet they are fun to make and therapeutic nonetheless.

Foot bath: Wrap a cluster of peppermint or lemon peel in cheesecloth and add to the hot water of a foot bath.

Room freshener: Add essential oils to pre-mixed potpourri.

Bathroom cleaner and freshener: Place 2 or 3 drops of oil on a wet cloth or sponge and place in the wash water. Oils that are recommended are lemon, bergamot, lavender, sweet orange, oregano or thyme.

To discourage colds in your home, add four to nine drops of the following to the water of a humidifier, or six drops per cup of water for a room spray: eucalyptus, thyme, rosemary, lemon or marjoram.

In the car, add three to six drops of oil to _ cup of baking soda and put the mixture in the empty car ashtray (obviously do not do this if you use the ashtray for ashes): peppermint, sweet orange, lavender, lemon or citronella.

As potpourri: Even small gardens, or those of friends and neighbors, can yield enough fragrant flowers and plants to create potpourri. For instance, highly fragrant roses such as Mister Lincoln and Double Delight, along with lavender, lemon verbena, cloves and cinnamon, can be the basis of a sweet treat for the senses. Here are some recipes I recommend. I'm a low-tech person and these are easy. Remember, you can improvise.

The mixing directions are all the same. All ingredients should be dried before combining, and you'll need a large bowl, a wooden spoon and, eventually, containers with tightly fitting lids if you plan to share the potpourri. After combining the ingredients, you'll want to let it rest for a few days in a container with a tightly fitting lid or in a sealed plastic bag. Label the product, and put it in a dark place so that the fragrances blend.

Potpourri should blend fragrances and textures. You might want to save and dry a few roses, slices of dried orange peel or even add some tiny shells to the final mixture. I like to see and feel chunks in the potpourri I've created, so I always include cinnamon sticks and slices of dried citrus peel.

Just Roses

2 handfuls of rose petals and buds

2 handfuls of rose geranium leaves

2 bay leaves crumbled

1 tablespoon vanilla extract

1 teaspoon orris (a fixative)

4 drops rose oil, an essential oil (optional)

Lavender Dreams

2 handfuls of lavender

1 handful of sweet marjoram

1 handful of rosemary

2 teaspoons ground allspice (pumpkin pie spice works, too)

2 teaspoons orris (fixative)

4 drops of lavender oil (optional)

Garden Bouquet

3 handfuls of garden flowers

1 handful fragrant leaves or sweet herbs, such as rosemary

1 handful mint

1 teaspoon of spice (your choice)

2 teaspoons orris (fixative)

4 drops of rose oil (optional)

Summer Zest

2 handfuls of garden flowers (including orange or lemon blossoms)

1 handful of sweet herbs or fragrant leaves

1 cup orange or lemon zest

1 handful basil

1 handful eucalyptus leaves

2 teaspoons orris (fixative)

1 teaspoon of your favorite spice

Smart gardeners, herbalists and experts on aromatherapy steer clear of any plants and flowers that have been sprayed with pesticide. Poisons cling to the flowers and leaves and are inhaled when you breathe in the fragrance. Definitely not a good thing. Instead, use the recipe for Bug Juice, a non-toxic bug repellent, in chapter 1. It can be used on your ingredients while they're still on the stalk, as long as you're not allergic to any of the juice's ingredients.

Some flowers and plants cause allergic reactions. Imagine giving a goldenrod allergy sufferer a potpourri of goldenrod. Yes, it'd be ugly. Your physician's advice and your own gardener's sense are well worth consulting on all natural therapies.

When mixing oils, only do so in glass containers, and label the mixtures. Store in a cool, dark place. Some people are highly allergic to oils, and experts warn against using them if you're pregnant, epileptic or have asthma, high blood pressure or sensitive skin. Essential oils are highly flammable and may stain fabric, carpets and wood. Just use common sense and be careful.

With all the rich history for this smell-good therapy, we must also be fair and listen to what contemporary medical practitioners have to say. Harley Goldberg, M.D., director of complementary and alternative medicine for Kaiser Permanente medical centers says, "The use of any therapy should be done with good common sense in conjunction with your total care. If stopping and smelling the roses feels good, it's a reasonable thing to do, just don't get caught in the thorns."

According to the *Journal of the American Medical Association* (November 11, 1998) "Trends in Alternative Medicine Use in the United States, 1990-1997," more adults are using complementary therapies than ever before. Between 1990 and 1997 (when the study was completed), there was nearly a 50 percent increase in visits and consultations by alternative medicine practitioners. That added up to more than 629 million visits during 1997, with a conservative price tag of about $21.2 billion.

The AMA is aware that Americans who visit providers and use alternative medical practices rarely disclose this information to their physicians. In the summary of the report, it's recommended that "Federal agencies, private corporations, foundations and academic institutions adopt a more proactive posture..." so that research and support can be given to complementary therapies, such as the use of fragrant plants and herbs.

As Dr. Dean Edell points out in *HealthCentral*, a report of alternative therapies, "Many users believe essential oils have the power to cure. That they're anti-bacterial, anti-viral and anti-fungal. But the scientific research just isn't there to back up such claims, which doesn't mean aromatherapy lacks benefits...until the research can prove it, healthy skepticism is a must." Dr. Edell and other medical advisors say that we can enjoy the relaxing effects of aromatherapy for that alone, yet if a claim sounds too good to be true, it probably is.

A fragrant garden with flowers in full bloom replenish our souls and sprits. Smells can influence our moods. But can they make us feel better?" As many gardeners know, the good can often come from sitting back and simply enjoying the relaxing effects of aromatherapy.

The good gardener commonly borrows his
methods, if not his goals, from nature herself.
– Michael Pollan, Second Nature

If you catch hold of the cat by its tail,
it will bite you. The world will do the same.
Live in the world like water on a lotus leaf.
—Yogaswami,
Positive Thoughts for Daily Meditation

Call Me Herb

Selecting herbs, preparing the soils for herbs, and growing herbs is gratifying and satisfying on lots of levels. It's a huge part of Nature's Health Plan at its best because you can eat the end results in salads, soups, or breads, among other things. You can make delicious herbal teas that are healthy and without the stimulants found in commercial brands. And breathing in the fragrance as you walk through your garden can be potent therapy to your mind.

Herbs go anywhere in the garden, and I think they are the queens and kings of the plant world. Once you master the easy tricks, you'll feel compelled to add them to your garden, if just for the fact that you can.

As part of your *Shovel It* program, think of herbs on the windowsill decorating the balcony and combined with flowers and vegetables. Think of adding herbs to garden containers, especially those straight outside the kitchen door, so that next time you're whipping up a zesty marinara, you can reach for some sprigs of rosemary and thyme and make that sauce sing.

Herbs are easy to grow regardless of where you live, especially if you're growing them indoors. Select the types that you'll actually use and enjoy, whether for tea, soup or decoration. Make sure that any herbs used in cooking, in cosmetics or that you put straight into your mouth from the garden are pesticide free. There are lots of non-toxic and effective bug repellents, such as the Bug Juice mentioned in chapter 1, that work well to keep herbs pest-free.

I love rosemary. It's hardy, fragrant, attractive and has luscious tiny, pale blue flowers. It's a no-fuss plant that withstands even forgetful gardeners like me. Not only do I cook with it, I smuggle long sprigs of rosemary within bunches of roses and feverfew, so that when friends drink in the perfume of the flowers, they get the soothing effect of this aromatherapeutic herb.

Speaking of therapy, herbs have a long, highly respected history in the medical field. Are you aware that about one-quarter of the prescription drugs ordered by physicians and dispensed by pharmacies here in the United States contain at least one active ingredient derived from plant material?

Although medicine seems like it has a solution for every ill, the World Health Organization estimates that 80 percent of the world's population, presently use herbal medicine for some aspect of health care.

Since the beginning of time and throughout all cultures, herbs, plants and plant materials have been used for folk medicine. In ancient times, people collected herbs for medical uses and had well-defined herbal pharmacopoeias. No one really knows when herbs were collected in the wild and then domesticated, but Egyptian records dating back to 2800 BC show herbs prescribed as medicine and used in food and in cosmetics, perfumes and dyes. Many herbs were thought to have magical powers. Even today in rural areas of Mexico, basil is sometimes carried in pockets to attract money. At one time ancient Scottish people drank tea made with thyme to prevent nightmares and to gain strength and courage.

Are you aware that Christopher Columbus was seeking a shorter route to India and those glorious spices, which were worth their weight in gold, when he bumped in to the Americas. Before Columbus, cinnamon, cloves, ginger, black pepper and other herbs came to Europe from Asia via overland caravans and were brought into ports such as Venice. The journey was long, fraught with various dangers and deprivation, and thus the prices for these precious ingredients skyrocketed.

The American Medical Association, in the *Journal of the American Medical Association*, November/December 1998, advises its members of the growing number of patients who use medicinal herbs, and to be aware that more of their patients will be doing so in the future. Many herbal cures hold promising results for diseases of today. In an Australian study conducted in 1998 and published in the *Journal of the American Medical Association*, it was revealed that a Chinese herbal medicine may help treat symptoms of irritable bowel syndrome. This is a condition that affects as many as one in five Americans and tends to respond poorly to conventional medical care. The blind study, discussed in "Chinese Herbs Soothe Irritable Bowel Syndrome" by A. Bensoussan and N.J. Talley, et al., indicates that a standard Chinese herbal pill containing licorice and ginger along with 20 other herbs, resulted in improvement in half of those taking the herbal formula. Less than a third of those taking placebos improved.

"More than one third of Americans use herbs for health purposes, yet patients often lack accurate information about the safety and efficacy of herbal remedies," writes MaryAnn O'Hara, M.D., and others in "A Review of 12 Commonly Used Medicinal Herbs." Before you treat yourself, loved ones or animal companions with any herbal remedy, whether you've found it on the Internet or the recipe has been passed down in your family, it's smart to talk with your doctor. Oftentimes herbal remedies counteract other medications, diminishing or reversing the effect of the prescription. Some long-time "cures" can be harmful for those with medical conditions or during pregnancy.

Here's the lowdown and lore on some of the more popular spices and herbs.

Basil: Used in sauces, salads and soups and to flavor vinegars in sixteenth century Europe. Lovers would exchange sprigs of basil as indications of their faithfulness. Some tales explain how if a woman gives a man basil and he accepts it, he'll fall in love with her and never leave. Indians used it to swear their oaths in court. Treasure hunters and gamblers have tried the Mexican tradition of carrying basil in their pockets to attract money.

Dill: The Egyptians used it in a tea form to soothe the body. Greeks used it to calm hiccups. In the Middle Ages, dill was the best way to repel witchcraft. Brought to the New World by those seeking religious freedom, dill seeds became known as "meetin' seed" because children would chew them during long sermons. And today some people still chew the seed to sweeten breath after a spicy meal.

Garlic: If you wanted to repel vampires, this was the herb you selected. In today's vampire-free society, it's the favorite herb grown by chefs and cooks, and it's easy to propagate. If you'd like to grow garlic, you can order the heads (as the bulbs are called, because they look much like a flower bulb) from seed companies and growers. While you won't be able to determine the variety, you can get fresh garlic at the grocery store, pull apart the bulb and separate the garlic cloves, then plant them. Be warned—it spreads. For flower lovers, the flowers of the garlic are lovely, tall spherical bursts that when left to mature and dry, add interest to fall arrangements. And no, they don't smell like garlic. Because garlic was thought to have magical qualities, it was used to cast spells and in charms. Some folklorists tell how garlic is used to absorb disease, and some people rub pots and pans with garlic to keep negative energies away from food. According to the American Medical Association in an article from the November/December 1998 journal, "Dozens of trials suggest, but have not adequately proven, that garlic can decrease the risk factors for arteriosclerosis, particularly hypercholesterolemia," and anecdotal claims that garlic has medical powers continue.

Mint: It's been used for thousands of years, and in Roman times was considered essential for hospitality. In Greek mythology, Minthe (sometimes referred to as Menthe) was a nymph adored by Pluto, who transformed her into this scented, unforgettable herb. There are more than 600 varieties of mint, the most common being peppermint and spearmint. All mints come with a warning if you live in a temperate climate. Once you plant it, it will not go away. Years ago, my mother shoveled spearmint out of a pot and into her barren garden, thinking it would decompose and help the soil. The next spring, even the lawn mower and tiller couldn't eradicate it. Unless you're okay about how the mint will take over, and I really mean take over, plant it in a pot or container. Some people place a pot of mint directly into the soil, but I've found that the mint sends out runners, those growing shoots, and in a blink of an eye, it's there in the garden. For good.

Spearmint and peppermint are used in love sachets in order to attract Mr. or Ms. Right, and folklorists say to carry mint in the pocket while traveling to protect oneself and for a safe journey home. It's also said to attract wealth, so you might want to put a sprig in your wallet or purse next time you're up for a raise. I like to make mint tea. It's fun, too, to freeze a few mint leaves in ice cubes to add to lemonade, juices and iced teas. It's commonly known to aid digestion, soothing a tummy after spicy foods or during the stomach flu, and may reduce heartburn and flatulence. A strong infusion or tea (say 3 cups of boiling water poured over 3 mint tea bags) makes a lovely, relaxing foot soak or can be added to a bath.

Oregano: This herb received its name from oros ganos or "joy of the mountain." It's an ancient herb, a symbol of happiness. It's also called wild marjoram. Today we commonly use it in pizza, Italian dishes and soups, but it was once rubbed over oak furniture and floors to protect the finish and add freshness to the house. Ancient Greeks used it as a remedy for poisoning, which is scary since there seems little scientific evidence to support this claim. Folklorists recommend making a tea with oregano leaves to counteract a nervous headache and to relieve seasickness.

Parsley: At one time it was thought that misfortune would befall you if a stranger came into your garden and planted parsley. Today, I for one would thank this person. Parsley is more than a garnish, it adds flavor, texture and colors to hundreds of dishes. The Greeks used it to weave into wreaths, and it was believed that Hercules chose parsley as his personal herb. It was also used in funeral rituals and to decorate tombs. The Romans continued the funerary practices but also brought it home to use as a Roman air freshener. It was lavishly included in the Roman feasts as part of the meal. Folklore specialists say that the herb should be eaten to promote fertility and fidelity, but I like it in soup, tuna salad, scrambled eggs, mashed potatoes and pasta dishes.

Thyme: Used by the Greeks to show graceful elegance, today it is a favorite among cooks. Roman soldiers used to bathe in thyme water to promote vigor. Egyptians used it as an antiseptic (it was also used this way during World War I) and as a method of preserving foods long before plastic zip bags and refrigeration were available. The ancient Scots used thyme tea to prevent nightmares and to gain strength and courage over their enemies. In addition to use in cooking, a thyme tea can be used as the final rinse to make hair more manageable. Folklorists say it can be used as a compress to reduce swelling from insect bites. Include a few drops of thyme essential oil in potpourri or in laundry rinse water to bring a lovely, fresh smell.

Here are some favorite herbs to use as tea. Again, only use those herbs that are organic and best yet, grown in your own planter boxes so you know they are pesticide free. You can also find these teas available at specialty stores and online.

Chamomile: Soothes nerves and calms the stomach.

Elderflower: Refreshing decongestant.

Lemon Verbena and Lemon Balm: Produces a lemonade flavor and lifts the spirits on a winter day.

Peppermint: Soothes upset stomach, reduces gas, and just makes you feel wonderful.

When the College of Physicians of Philadelphia was founded in 1787, Benjamin Rush, M.D., proposed a garden of medicinal herbs to be planted "to physick the citizens of Philadelphia." Today you can still visit the oasis, the Medicinal Herb Garden, which is open to the public six days a week. Rush, a signer of the Declaration of Independence, has been called the father of American psychiatry for his systematic description of mental illness and its treatment and for improving the care of the mentally ill. Herbalists thank him for seeing herbal and homegrown medicines as an essential part of his practice.

With all the strong, continued interest in herbs and herbal medicine, doctors and health care providers must talk with their patients about complementary therapies. As a suggestion, medical advisors might want to remember that not so long in the past, when someone had a headache, a piece of willow bark was torn from the tree, boiled in water, strained and the liquid drunk. This was the forebear of aspirin. Herbal medicine isn't going away, nor will the medical professionals, and it's time to work together for the best of the patient.

One must never look for happiness:
one meets it by the way...
—Isabelle Eberhardt, author
and English adventurer (1877-1904)

*The goal of your life is living
in agreement with nature.*
—Zeno

Coping's A Big Garden Job

Shovel It, deal with it, and find ways to cope. Yes, you can cope with life when you have a handle on how to do it. No, it's not easy, nor is it fair. Grandmother may have said, "Life's no walk in the park." I like to add that it's no walk in the garden, either. Whether you have scars from working in a rose garden or have overcome or coped with tragedy in life, that adage rings true.

Coping is a learned skill. For unfathomable reasons, it comes easier to some humans than others. Here are some tips to make this garden job a bit easier.

❁ Identify stressors, the things that ruffle your feathers or send you off the edge. Knowing beforehand that you're expected to host the summer's best party, even though you hate the idea, could be the ticket to sleepless nights and a nervous twitch. Once you pinpoint stressors you can make decisions on how you'll deal with them. You might still have to host the party, but how about doing it in the park, if you don't want the nieces, nephews and an assortment of kids to trample your clematis, campanula and coreopsis.

❀ Be sensitive to your body and what it says. Don't ignore pain or discomfort. If you're having trouble sleeping or coping with issues, talk to your doctor. If she or he isn't able to listen to you, find someone else.

❀ Practice deep breathing.

❀ Use garden exercise, yoga, aromatherapy and herbal teas to create ways to lower your stress.

❀ If you don't like what your body, mind or spirit is telling you, consult with your medical professional or a listening friend. The alternative is to be out of control, and that's dangerous, weed-infested ground indeed.

❀ Smile and practice smiling. Do this while you're alone, especially if you haven't had much to smile about lately. Yes, smiling might take some practice.

❀ Approach stressful events with a positive attitude. Stop focusing on the problem and look around for help and ways to figure out a solution. If you know you're going to be late for a meeting because traffic is tied up for miles, call and explain the situation. Reschedule the meeting, or use the time to go over how you'll supply solutions.

❀ Understand that if you're grieving, whether for the end of a dream or the death of a loved one, you are going through mental and physical changes. Feelings of loss are caused by feelings of love. During the process of grief, everyone experiences five stages, yet it's valuable to note that they rarely occur in a set pattern. The stages are denial, anger, bargaining, depression and acceptance. When researching and interviewing for my book on death and grief, *What to Do When a Loved One Dies*, and then lecturing nationwide on the topic, I found time and again that most Americans are scared to death of death. Most don't want to talk about it; few prepare for it. We must remember during any period of change, whether it's facing a death or moving away from a perfect garden, perfect house and perfect community, that it's okay to cry, to question, to be weak. Grief is an active process. Freud rightly labeled it work because it is mental and physical labor. It's exhausting, not only for the bereaved but for those around you who try to comfort and also cope. No two people work through grief in the same way, and children, the disabled and older adults often grieve silently because they are unable to express their emotions. But grief and death are a natural part of living, and just like the seasons of the year, the cycle continues.

❀ Be a learner and gain new perspective from each of life's events and hurdles. Be wise enough to change what you can, accept that which you cannot change and to know the difference between the two.

❀ Ask for help. Close personal relationships are our life preservers in a tumultuous sea. If you do not have this support from your family, and many of us do not, then begin to form new connections now with others within your church, synagogue, civic organization, group or a club. Share your load and allow prayer and meditation to be part of your solution to coping. If problems in life come to the point where you cannot see any light at the end of any tunnel, waste no time. Consult with a listening friend, your clergy and/or a therapist. Bereavement groups, often sponsored by hospice and hospital programs, allow those who are attempting to cope find help in a group situation with a leader who is experienced with the job of coping. It's good to let off steam and share the load.

❀ Reinvent yourself. Try new things. Dress, eat and act in other ways. Wear a hot pink shirt. Cut your hair. Grow a beard. Plant bearded iris. Remove all the grass and plant a meadow. Learn to paint murals so you can decorate the garden fence. Join clubs. Revise who you are so that the new you can survive. After any gut-wrenching experience, you are different. I compare it to how our grandparents mended holes in socks. When I get a hole, I walk to the trash can, drop the sock in and say, "Darn." Paulina, my maternal grandmother, would be scandalized by my darning method. She expertly used a needle and thread for this process. But even the best-skilled needle person couldn't totally conceal where the hole had once been. It's the same with a broken heart. The crack or hole is always there, but by finding new ways of living, we can mend it well enough to continue to live.

❀ Get organized. Finish a gardening task you've been putting off for a long time.

❀ Try getting rid of clutter. Throw out or give away things that do not make you happy or do not bring you joy, unless it's unlawful to do so. Throw out or give away things that you do not enjoy looking at. Add to this pile things that you haven't used in a year, unless there's good sentimental attachment. Just because someone gives you a present, it doesn't mean you must keep it. Someone dear recently gave me a few Depression-era plates, "When I saw these, I knew they'd be perfect for dessert," she said in the note. Yes, they were darling, and I loved them and really appreciated her thoughtfulness. Then I passed them on to my sister. She'll use them. They'd just collect dust in the back of a cupboard for me because I'm not the delicate, expensive china type hostess.

❀ Realize that few things are irreplaceable, except legal documents, photos (including those from when Fido was a pup), and your children's drawings and the other stuff that they made in elementary school. If you have given away a gardening guide and realize it too late, you'll surely be able to track down another.

❀ Avoid harmful coping devices such as smoking, drinking or drugs. Nicotine stimulates the release of adrenaline and the stress hormone cortisol. This increases heart rate, elevates blood pressures, causes sweating and increases nervousness. Excessive caffeine keeps the body in a state of perpetual alarm. It speeds the heart rate and induces the stress/anxiety symptoms from headache, insomnia, upset stomach and sweaty palms all the way to ulcers.

❀ Create nighttime rituals so that you can get a good night's sleep. Try to go to bed at the same time each evening so that your body gets used to a pattern. Keep the bedroom a work-free and television-free zone.

❀ Put on your garden shoes and get outdoors. Regular exercise can have longer-lasting benefits than taking antidepressant medication, according to a study in *Psychosomatic Medicine* (September 29, 2000) as conducted by researchers from Duke University Medical Center, North Carolina. The results of the study showed that when motivated people continue to exercise, they have a much better chance than non-exercising and motivated people to never see their depression return. The *Journal of the American Medical Association* supports this thesis with a physical twist. In the April 12, 1999, Journal, Rozenn N. Lemaitre, Ph.D., MPH, and others write, "The results [of the study and research] suggest that regular participation in moderate-intensity activities, such as walking and gardening, are associated with a reduced risk of PCA [primary cardiac arrest]." In the study this life-saving information was based on only 60 minutes of gardening each week. Gardening is THAT powerful and could save lives.

❀ Write down what's up. Use your garden journal or start a personal journal to sketch out what's eating at you and to discover how better to cope. Don't share the journal. As a matter of fact, hide it well. This is for your eyes only. If you're tossing and turning, keep a notepad by your bed, write down the problem, and often in the morning the answer will miraculously appear. You'll find more on journaling and photo journals by consulting the index.

❀ Talk and spend time with others. Sure, there are garden clubs where it's more important to see what type of car you drive than to determine what disease is attacking your Rose Cushion phlox, but they're on the wane. Most newspapers have a weekly listing of sociation, so if you're nuts for a specific type of plant, vegetable or flower, you'll surely find others who are, too. You can find plant chat rooms online if you'll hunt around a bit, or you can start one of your own.

❀ Keep your work life and non-work life and problems separate. This is tough if you have, like I do, an office in the home. But really now, that's what doors are for.

❀ Stop procrastinating. When it comes to a difficult or painful task, just get to it. *Shovel It* out of your life. Putting things off only makes them more trying.

❀ Take a mini-vacation. Lie under a tree, do the stretching exercises found in chapter 5, begin writing in your garden journal and take a trip to the garden center.

❀ Learn to breathe for your health's sake. Participate in regular exercise. Get outdoors for sunshine, a walk and definitely working in the garden.

❀ Move toward a simple life. Pay or barter with others for child care or adult care, learn to delegate, get good at managing time. Turn off the television or record your favorite programs. Turn off the phone or the pager and don't check your office e-mail on the weekend. Spend an hour of time, at the minimum, just on you. This isn't easy, and trust me, you'll find a zillion excuses why you can't spend time on yourself. But once you make this a habit, you'll feel like you've had a recess from life; it's addictive and good for you.

❀ When you feel your coping skills fading and you're in a safe place (not driving down the interstate), try this: Don't move a muscle. Look only where you can see without turning your head. Look closely at anything that interests you. See something weird or unusual? Focus on that. Use this image to trigger a happy memory, find a solution, fantasize or daydream about an adventure or person or place. Take a few deep breaths and relax.

❀ Meditate or pray while holding a flower, blade of grass or piece of wood. Touch the object, smell it, brush it against your cheek. Ask Nature or God to direct your mind to a peaceful solution or a time of rest. Relax. Give it time.

❀ *Shovel It.*

> The ultimate lesson all of us have to learn
> is unconditional love, which includes not only
> others but ourselves as well.
> —Elisabeth Kubler-Ross, author,
> grief expert

Chapter 7

Share Power
in the Garden

*Blackberry winter, the time when hoarfrost
lies on the blackberry blossoms; without this
frost the berries will not set. It is the
forerunning of a rich harvest.*
—Margaret Mead, anthropologist

Your garden might be a few pots of herbs on the doorstep or humongous expanses planted to near perfection to take one's breath away. If that's the case, I'm jealous and coming over to see how you do it all. Where, when and how you garden matters little because you can have the same healthy, therapeutic pleasures even if you find them in the abundant public gardens and green areas around the world. For instance, it is possible to have a garden party, even if your garden is on the windowsill or at the community park.

I love sharing my garden and hosting yearly Rose Parties at the height of my rose garden's beauty, which is any time between mid-April and June. Keep in mind that my garden will never be mistaken for one in the fancy landscaping magazines. It's comfortable and whimsical. In the springtime it's chock full of flowers, which makes up for any blemish. While my parties are far from something everyone's Auntie May might host, they are fun, and a good time is always had by all.

On a Saturday afternoon in May, neighbors, friends, family, colleagues and those people I meet all the time at the post office, library and church come over. Everyone wears Saturday clothes. Grubbies. You know the ones: jeans, shorts, T-shirts and sneakers. The food? You'll find some recipes here in this chapter that are quick, painless to make, even for non-gourmet cooks, and they'll certainly impress your friends and loved ones. At least they do with my friends and loved ones, but perhaps these folks are just easily razzle-dazzled.

I like simple entertaining. One year I served sparkling water still in their fancy blue bottles. I bought a few pounds of decadent chocolate. The day of the party, I loaded up on the most humongous apple-sized strawberries I could find. Tableware? Paper cups, paper napkins. It was a huge success, and friends now pester me for the date of the next party.

I could have waited until the garden was perfect and the house was finished being remodeled and my hands healed from pulling weeds and the moon was finally found to be made of green cheese. Or do as I do and share the health-restoring and therapy-providing experience of being in the garden.

Can a garden party really help people who aren't feeling up to snuff? If hospitalized patients' wounds heal faster and they require fewer painkillers and fewer antidepressants when merely looking at a painting of a garden, imagine the effect your garden can have. Imagine the effects of visiting, sitting in and having a party in one that's real, that's live. That's a small reason why Joseph, my husband, and I have garden parties. Another is that we love to, and it makes us happy.

Sometimes it's fun to play games, even with grown-ups, and you'll soon find some I've enjoyed. I especially like old-fashioned scavenger hunts. Why, you may want to hand gardening guests clippers so that they can pick their own bouquet to take home. If you're well organized, you could have a potpourri party with the recipes you'll find in this book, and regardless of the weather outdoors, each guest can return home with a breath of summer.

A few years ago I was part of a progressive garden party. We started at one friend's garden, carpooled to another, and so forth, until in one afternoon we'd visited six different rose gardens, ending at my home for a feast of potluck desserts. Some of the gardens were three rose bushes along a front path and others were elaborate and should have come from *Country Living* magazine. Not only did we see each other's gardens at their best, but we shared plants and seeds and cuttings. You might say we bonded with chunks of regal geraniums (sometimes referred to as Martha Washington geraniums), bulbs, sunflowers (in seeds) and plenty of cuttings.

All it takes to host a garden party and to share your garden is creativity. That's what *Shovel It* is all about, finding ways to honor our creative selves.

That's the focus of this chapter: ways to share your garden and encourage others with Nature's Health Plan. You'll find garden parties with recipes and ways to share your bounty. If you're interested in photographing your garden and want to know the reasons why it could make you feel better, you'll find it in this chapter. Here, too, you might decide it's past time to let your garden go to the birds and gather even more therapy with these creatures loving your part of the planet. As always, the choices in the garden and your *Shovel It* therapy are yours.

Nature never forces you to punch a time clock.

Make-believe colors the past with innocent
distortion, and it swirls ahead of us
in a thousand ways—in science,
in politics, in every bold intention.
It is part of our collective lives, entwining
our past and our future...a particularly
rewarding aspect of life itself.
—Shirley Temple Black

Adam was a gardener, and God,
who made him, sees that half of all good
gardening is done upon the knees.
—Rudyard Kipling, author

It's Party Time

If gardening makes you feel great, imagine what it will do for friends, family, neighbors and co-workers. It's blissful to share your garden if you don't obsess over having everything apple-pie perfect. If you try to achieve perfection, you'll only diminish the joy and therapy. Only God creates perfection. We mortals never achieve it. Get a grip and deal with your humanity.

That's right: It's party time.

Just for the sake of getting a bit of exercise, walk around your garden right now. You can take this book, too. Feel how therapeutic it is to breathe in the fragrances of spring or summer. It's fall? Drink in the glorious colors. Such reds, those russets, and just look at the yellow. Practically need to squint sometimes, don't you, because it's so bright. And in the winter there's a feeling of potential under a layer of snow or leaves. Can you sense the tulips and daffodils still snuggled down under a thick layer of mulch and the richness of the soil waiting for you to acknowledge their presence? What a lovely feeling of anticipation. It's much like being a kid counting the days until Christmas, isn't it?

Don't hesitate. A garden party is simple. Try to choose a time and date when you can have guests come and go, indoors and out without rain. You may want to include a rain date on the invitation so you don't have to call 50 people if the weather suddenly changes on the day of the event. Most gardeners like to hold the party between 2:00 and 5:00 in the afternoon, the traditional teatime, because there's a lot of flexibility in what you can serve. You can make or buy finger sandwiches and scones, veggies and dip. Blending low-fat yogurt loaded with herbs is a great one for calorie-counting gardeners. This, too, might be the time to take down Grandmother's silver service or the china teapot you've never used, and set an elegant outdoor table for the party. Plates are optional at finger-food parties, but napkins are a necessity.

You may want to serve teas, including herbal teas made from peppermint or lemon verbena harvested in your own garden. Here's a simple recipe for Chamomile Tea. Of course, never make tea, sandwiches or even potpourri from plants, flowers or herbs that have been treated with pesticides or insecticides.

Garden Chamomile Tea

Warm a teapot. Add about 1 cup of crushed, dried chamomile flowers. You'll want to experiment with this recipe before the party to make sure you like the strength of the tea. Pour boiling water over the herb and allow to steep for five minutes. Sweeten with honey or sugar.

You can use the same recipe for peppermint and lemon verbena tea.

At some garden parties, only sherry, champagne, wine or the finest sparkling waters can make the magic complete. Many party stores have plastic, recyclable glassware that looks like it should hold champagne. Children love fancy dress-up parties, and you may want to suggest that everyone come in costume with huge hats, flowing gowns, loads of jewelry and pretend that you're all back in Victorian times.

For those who come without the prerequisite outfit, have long strings of beads and bobbles and gaudy hats available at the garden gate.

Here's a recipe for cucumber sandwiches that'll please even the serious sandwich eaters. You can add to the filling with thin slices of zesty cheese or salami, or go over the edge and use caviar. For those with delicate sensibilities, trim off the bread crusts and serve on lace doily covered plates or silver platters:

Cucumber Tea Sandwiches with Tarragon Butter

1 large English cucumber or cucumber from your garden, scrubbed, peeled, sliced
   paper thin

1/2 teaspoon salt

2 tablespoons white vinegar

1 cup unsalted butter, softened

1/4 cup minced fresh tarragon

1/4 cup minced fresh chervil

30 thin slices whole-wheat bread, enough to make 60 (2 x 4 inch rectangles)

Watercress leaves (optional)

Put cucumber slices in large bowl. Toss with salt. Sprinkle with vinegar.

Toss mix well. Let stand 1 hour. Drain well in colander.

Combine butter, tarragon and chervil.

To assemble, spread butter over 1 side of each bread slice.

Cover 15 slices with cucumbers, dividing evenly. Close sandwiches. Trim crusts.

Cut into 30 rectangles. Arrange on platter, garnished with watercress leaves.

It's game time. Here are some games nearly guaranteed to put zip into your garden party.

If you have a large garden or are holding your party in a public garden or community park, a scavenger hunt is exciting for all ages. When there are guests younger than 10, I recommend that they be partnered with a teenager or adult, and, of course, safety should always be a top priority when children are in public areas. Just create a long list of discoveries for each guest to make and/or collect.

Don't want the bearded iris defrocked or lemon tree stripped of all its fruit? Designate what players must do when they discover the plant. For instance, perhaps players must count the lemons on the branch tied with a red ribbon, or the number of pink bearded iris in a bed full of purple ones, and then add the number to the list.

Depending on the players, make the game simple ("Find five red leaves") to difficult ("List the types of rudbeckia").

You may want to give clues rather than a list, or even have a treasure hunt with a prize at the end, such as a well-wrapped box of bulbs or a garden tool. With children, I like to make sure everyone wins. Offer all the children first prizes, and give packets of seeds or potted tomato plants.

Another game is to design a garden hat. Provide or have each guest bring an old baseball cap and a glue gun. When working with children, you'll want to have an older child or adult supervise the gluing. On a covered picnic table, buy or save a variety of dried flowers and herbs, grasses that look like squirrel's tails, tiny cones, nuts, twigs and seedpods. Provide fresh flowers, too, that will last a few hours; you'll want to experiment to find those that work best in your area. The object of the game is to design the silliest, weirdest, wildest or most attractive garden hat. Create a party atmosphere and always applaud loudly for everyone's endeavors.

Think Hawaii in January and hand out the poi. Pretend to be in Anchorage in July and serve baked Alaska. Scour websites and magazines for zany party ideas, use ethnic finger-food recipes and dream up childhood games for the adults in your family. Invite neighbors, the couple down the street you don't know well but your kids play together, your music teacher, the preacher and her family, and your own loved ones (or they'll have a fit). Then let the fun begin as you share your garden's therapy.

> It seems to me we can never give up
> longing and wishing while we are alive.
> There are certain things we feel to be
> beautiful, and we must hunger for them.
> —George Eliot, author

Manners are a sensitive awareness of the feelings of others. If you have that awareness, you have good manners, no matter what fork you use.
—Emily Post, etiquette expert and author

Sharing Your Bounty

About five years ago, I planted a pony pack of Sweet 100 cherry tomatoes. Tiny plants, they were, when I picked them out at the nursery, but not for long. They have a reputation for mass-producing the tastiest treats on the Planet Earth. We love tomatoes of any shape or form, and I was actually worried that itinerant, marauding bunnies might eat the seedlings before they matured.

Apparently the bunnies found other delights in my garden, such as roses, because I had a bumper crop of Sweet 100s. Eventually, even the neighbors wouldn't come to the front door when they saw me approaching with a bowl of plump, red miniature tomatoes. I could see the curtains close when I walked up a driveway. Colleagues rudely declined offers after I forced on them the first, second and third avalanches. I have no evidence, but I think relatives started screening phone calls. If you've ever had a bumper crop of anything, you know that sooner, more than later, you need to reach out to others, or the crop goes to waste. That spells heartbreak for the gardener.

There are many ways to share your bounty and your garden. We've talked about garden parties as one way. Now it's time to take Nature's Health Plan a step further. Here are some practical ways to share the goodness:

- ❀ Contact the local women's shelter, homeless shelter, or AIDS home. Ask if you'd be permitted to bring pesticide-free produce for their residents. Is there a Salvation Army center in your town? Along with churches and other worship centers, the Salvation Army staff often knows of families who need produce, a visit with flowers or someone to tend a garden.

- ❀ Call the hospital, care facility, Alzheimer's center and find out if you can donate flowers or potted plants.

- ❀ Take a bouquet of flowers to your neighbors, the vet, your physician, your insurance agent and the receptionist at work, and don't forget your hairdresser. He or she would love some, too.

- ❀ Visit a senior center and ask about giving classes on potpourri or flower arranging.

- ❀ Look in the phone book, and then make the call to any organization that uses volunteers. Explain how you and Nature want to help. Be creative with solutions.

- ❀ Create a meditation herb garden or decorative garden at your house of worship or the neighborhood YMCA or recreation center. Many hospitals now have gardens for patients, visitors and staff members to relax and revitalize after being in the stressful environment indoors. The Friendship and the Magical Gardens at Children's Hospital and Health Center in San Diego was created out of love for parents and their children.

- ❀ Talk to the people on your school board or at the local boys and girls clubs to find out if there's a need for a community or education garden that would fit in with a science/biology curriculum, one that studies bugs, insects, soils, birds and animals of the garden. Volunteer your time and encourage young lives to adopt a garden lifestyle that may stay with them forever.

❀ Join a gardening club.

❀ Get together with other plant lovers and have a plant sale from the cuttings, seeds, and plants from your garden. Sell organic fruits and vegetables. Donate the money to a worthwhile cause.

❀ Take classes in horticultural therapy and learn more about sharing the gift of your garden and gardening self.

You cannot hope to build a better world without improving the individuals. To that end each of us must work for his own improvement, and at the same time share a general responsibility for all humanity, our particular duty being to aid those to whom we think we can be most useful.
—Marie Curie (1867-1934)

...As they share the produce of the work
with people less fortunate economically,
patients picture themselves,
often for the first time, as productive
members of society.
—Dr. Will Menninger, Menninger
Foundation, Topeka, Kansas

Creating a Therapy Garden at a Facility

Horticultural therapy is a field just now being considered appropriate to be added to the courses at many colleges and universities. If you have a desire or goal to create a public therapy garden, your first step will be to explain and show the administration or board the benefits of a garden and how it can continue, even when you're no longer involved. As the saying goes, "Make a plan and work a plan."

Those who are credentialed or have learned through trial and error recommend keeping these things in mind if you plan to incorporate *Shovel It: Nature's Health Plan* into educational, institutional or hospital programs:

❀ Consider the abilities of the individuals in the program, their special needs, interests and limitations. Encourage participants to discover individual ways to engage in the garden; not all will have the same level of interest.

❀ Organize projects into groups where those with more abilities or stronger interests can encourage others.

❀ Organize the garden so that participants do most of the work. You may have to rethink ideas of perfect gardens and well-defined flower and vegetable beds. With this method, each participant will gain more from the program than having everything done for her or him.

❀ Avoid giving busy work. Plan the projects so that participants feel that they are needed.

❀ Attempt projects that can be completed in a small amount of time, a short-term goal, and discuss how these projects will all work together for the garden.

❀ If working in a flower or vegetable garden, decide how the products of the garden will be used, i.e., to share the produce with needy families or to give bouquets to those in nursing facilities or to the patients who cannot leave their rooms.

❀ Bring in speakers who understand your audience and share movies, videos, and gardening catalogs and magazines with participants. If you contact companies which sell seeds and plants to ask for a few extra copies of their catalogs for your participants, most will lavish you with booklets.

❀ Have participants keep journals or begin a photo journal of your project. You'll find information on garden journals by checking in the index and help on garden photo journals in this chapter.

❀ Don't award prizes for prize-winning plants or flowers, but for participation in the program. Give positive and honest feedback. Be genuine and lavish with consistent praise. Encouragement should be more generously applied than water or fertilizer to the plants.

❀ Talk with parents, caregivers, teachers and staff members about the healthy benefits of gardening, as discussed throughout the book.

❀ Delegate. You need not do everything yourself.

> If one is lucky, a solitary fantasy can totally transform one million realities.
> —Maya Angelou

The highest wisdom is kindness.
—The Gemara, The Talmud

Birds Galore

Birds brighten up the most dreary days. Some of them shout for joy. Robins lighten almost any mood. Any demanding scrub jay can make you laugh at that "me" attitude.

Sharing your garden can be done in hundreds of ways, and many find that one of their favorites is to create a sanctuary for birds. Whether you live in Manhattan, New York, or Manhattan, Kansas, or Manhattan Beach, California, or any place in between, you can attract birds to your garden and enjoy the ever-changing tableau of nature.

I know that in some parts of the country, crows are really objectionable, but in my suburban garden, they are a riot. Just the other day, I saw a family of four feasting on some leftover popcorn. We've had a visiting peacock (really), a transient quail (whom we named Dan), and lots of migratory birds who see our garden and consider it a bunch better than Club Med. We keep the binoculars and a book to identify western birds near the patio, so when strange feathered friends stop by, we know what we've got.

According to bird experts, formally known as ornithologists, there's never been a shorter supply of safe habitats for birds. Blame it on urban and suburban sprawl or a zillion other things, the point, of course, is that your garden can become a sanctuary for God's creatures. Designing gardens that attract birds will add to the stress-relieving prescription of your garden, and the birds benefit, too.

You must make a pledge when you decide to share your garden with birds not to use pesticides and insecticides. I've heard too many horror stories of accidents where the birds die and the gardeners feel terrible. Most birds eat spiders, caterpillars, some butterflies and even the poisoned grain you may stick down a gopher hole. If you spray for bugs, you're actually offering birds a poisoned food supply.

You'll also want to discourage predators that threaten birds. If Fluffy, your cat, is prone to stalking birds, keep the bird feeder high off the ground and in a place where kitty can't mosey on over for a snack.

The third decision is to realize that gardens that attract birds are never in perfect order. Since that's the way Nature really wants it, you may have to lower your gardening standards at least in one area of your garden. For instance, the less you rake beneath bushes, the better it is for the birds.

Birds have basic needs if you want them in your *Shovel It* garden: food, water and shelter. Even in winter they'll need these things since not all birds take a trip south to a sunny clime. When deciding to create a garden to share with birds, you'll need to be committed to providing these components. Here in my temperate Southern California garden, fresh water is the most important component of our bird-infested backyard. There are bugs and seeds and shelter provided by the mock orange bushes that line one side of the backyard, but it's the birdbath that they flock to. Yes, Joseph and I feed the birds, and we make sure that they have plenty of water.

Some people hang a plastic bottle of water with a hole in the bottom over their birdbath. Dripping water is like a magnet to birds. It drips and they come. Try it.

You can buy or build plain or fancy nesting boxes, birdhouses and feeders to entice the bird population. Stores and websites abound that offer pricey ones as well as those especially for limited budgets. You may want to consult with a bird guide for your area to make sure that the house you choose will be appropriate for those birds in your area.

Look around your garden for places where birds can hide and find shelter. Birds like thickets, dense shrubs and conifers, especially those which provide berries and seeds. You may want to leave some dead limbs or an entire dead tree standing, unless it is dangerous, to attract insects on which your feathered buddies can feast. Tunneling insects that live beneath rotting tree bark are an important food source for birds such as chickadees, woodpeckers and nuthatches. Since hollow trees are becoming extremely rare in our civilized world, cavity-nesting birds, such as bluebirds and woodpeckers, are finding it increasingly difficult to acquire nest sites.

Why not give your Christmas tree a new life and make winter birds deliriously happy. It's easy. After you "move" Christmas from the house, put the tree in a part of the garden where birds can have privacy. That is, don't stick it right where the kids want to skateboard or toss a ball. Within the branches, tie clusters of wheat or even the strings of popcorn you put together when the tree was indoors. Slices of fruit, such as apples and oranges will be appreciated. Fill pinecones with peanut butter and tie them onto the tree. If you want to get fancy, roll the peanut butter-filled pinecone in birdseed and then place it on the tree. When spring comes and the birds have more shelter as trees leaf out, simply discard or compost your bird tree. You can also buy conifers or spruce trees at the nursery for this purpose, but remember, you'll have to check the soil and pot size often to make sure that the tree is happy.

How about putting in a "condo" for birds? One made of dead branches will look like an uptown address to God's creatures. It'll give protection from the elements and from predators. Start the brush pile by placing thick branches in a stack about 2 feet deep. Then just place a few lighter ones on top. You'll have to add more as time progresses. You may want to place conifer branches or any other light greenery over the stack. This is a great project to share with the kids, but be sure to share that birds are shy and need to have their space.

What might look messy to Miss Manners is a 5-star resort to the birds. Keep some of the garden unkempt, even if it's only a small area at the back of your lot.

As you consider the plan of your garden and how you might share it with birds, talk with a tree expert at your local nursery for those tress that grow best in your climate zone.

A fun way to further experience your bird-filled garden is by keeping a birding journal, where garden birds are identified and the sighting is dated. Loved ones who are confined to the house or in a care facility especially love bird watching. First acquire a good book about birds, keep it and a pair of binoculars handy and you're in business. You might want to join a group of bird enthusiasts, too, or refer to one of many books on birds and gardens.

> Gardeners, I think,
> dream bigger dreams than emperors.
> —Mary Cantwell, gardener and author

*A little garden, the littler the better, is your
richest chance for happiness and success.*
—Reginald Farrer, author

You're So Photogenic

Remember that day last spring when you walked around your garden or a public garden and thought, "Wow, wouldn't that make a great photo." The colors, the textures and the lushness of it all made your heart go pitter pat. We've all felt that way. Smart gardeners rush inside and grab a camera. Most admit the photos never do justice; however, they are an excellent way to compare one year to the next and to recall memories.

So why not photograph your garden? Even amateur photos (trust me, that's what mine tend to be), provide a visual log that goes well beyond memories. These photos will boost spirits in the middle of February on one of those endlessly frozen afternoons.

Lots of gardeners create photo memory books along with their garden journal. In the photo memory book, gardeners describe the plant or flower in the photo and then write bits about what's going on in their lives at that time. You need not be an expert writer or photographer (yes, I needed to say that again), because this pictorial history of your garden can be for your eyes only.

Others photograph their garden and take photos when touring public gardens in order to share the pictures with family, friends and, heck, anyone who'll look at them. Photographing your garden might mean that loved ones in care centers can visit your garden without leaving their rooms. The photos of your garden might help with a loved one's recovery because, as we've talked about, just viewing a garden, even in a painting or a photograph, has been scientifically proven to decrease the need for pain medication and antidepressants in hospital patients.

Why, you might find that you enjoy garden photography so much you'll want to frame and perhaps show your work, create photo montages or add to your income by selling the photos or by making greeting cards.

Here's a basic course, titled Garden Photography 101.

It's the gospel truth: I'm not Ansel Adams, but many of my photos have been published right beside gardening, health and wellness articles. Did I just hear you say, "How can that be?" Let me explain.

Rethink about how you envision a roll of film. Those photos that turn out badly should be tossed out, thrown away. Do not keep the uglies among the keepers. No need to. A friend and excellent photographer, CeCe Cantón (who took the photo of me on the cover of this book) takes two rolls of film to get one great exposure. If that's how professionals do it, then we need to revise the snap-and-be-satisfied-with-it philosophy. I now follow the more-is-better technique because if it's good enough for CeCe, it's great for me.

I have a simple point-and-shoot camera. It's old, but it's easy to operate and lightweight. Choose one you can comprehend and tote around, too. Another friend loves camera equipment and he carries a huge bag of lenses, equipment, filters and other special stuff, of which I have no clue how to use. All that equipment is just too heavy and too much trouble for me.

Consumer Reports magazine often has informational articles on cameras, if you're in the market for a new one. The digital cameras are coming down in price, too, so if you're planning to create websites or send digital photos to family and friends, this might be the direction to take.

Your local library or video store probably has a "how to take better pictures" video to rent. I found them to be most helpful and before I toured Finland a few years ago, I watched one video three times so that I could make sure I understood the concepts and could apply them. You might also want to take a photography class at your community college or senior center, especially if you're planning on developing your own film.

Be sure to keep track of what you've snapped. While touring the gardens in Pennsylvania recently, I put coded stickers with numbers on the exposed film and then wrote in a journal the exposure number and location. For instance, when I was at the incredible Longwood Gardens, it was a perfect September day, unlike any we get in San Diego. It was deliciously cool in the morning shade and mellow in the sun. There wasn't a rain cloud in sight, although the rain from the night before made everything sparkle. As I walked through the lush surroundings, my trigger finger clicked and clicked and clicked. I only stopped to change rolls of film.

But what if I didn't follow my plan to keep track of what I'd photographed? I would return home, develop the film and, Oops! Now which orchid was that? Which palm is that? What building was that? You get the picture (pun intended). Keep notes of each photo or roll of photos.

If it's been a long time since you've used your camera, get it cleaned. I just did that. It cost about $25, and my old point-and-shoot camera is better than ever.

What should you avoid in photos? Susan McCartney, author of *Travel Photography* says, "Garbage." McCartney is talking about throwaway trash. I take this concept further. I believe any extras that diminish the focus or story that your photo is telling is garbage. For instance, let's say you're taking a snapshot of children and a golden retriever frolicking on the lawn with a backdrop of head-high sunflowers and marigolds nearing perfection, so bright you practically need sunglasses to look at them.

Picture it: Darling kids smiling broadly, happy blond dog, stunning day, emerald grass and those dazzling sunflowers with heads that are 18 inches in diameter. You look through the viewfinder. Yuck. There in the distance is also a grubby wheelbarrow and what was once a chew toy for the pooch. While the wheelbarrow might work, the chew toy is garbage. Check your viewfinder before you snap, but definitely look around to get the garbage out before you begin to take pictures.

Hold your breath while you snap any picture. It's one thing to stay very still, but by holding your breath as you click the picture, you'll always get better quality.

If you plan to sell your photos and you're taking photos of people, you'll need to get a photo release (unless you're taking crowd pictures). The release can be a simple, written statement giving you permission to use the photo in conjunction with your article or book. You should not be expected to pay to take someone's photo, but this has happened occasionally.

Keep in mind as you travel and tour gardens worldwide, in some cultures and countries it's considered extremely bad manners to take someone's picture without permission. Be aware of customs before you snap a shutter. When I was visiting New Mexico's Pueblo Taos, last year, a special photo permit had to be purchased if I wanted to take pictures of the Native American dwellings.

As you take photos, be aware that the image doesn't start with the camera; it ends there. When the shutter is released, the picture is recorded, for better or worse. To get the best picture, envision your choices before you let the camera take over. Ask these questions: Why am I taking the picture? What special significance does this person or place have? What makes the situation unusual? What mood do I want to achieve? What do I want people to see in the picture?

The questions and your answers will help produce better results.

Photography "sees" in two dimensions. Train yourself to view the world as the camera does. Hold your hands up to focus a frame around the object of your photo. Imagine the scene as if it were in a book. Does the image look lively? If it's dull, try moving to another angle. To convey size, add something or somebody to your composition to show the scale, such as those children playing in the foreground as the gigantic sunflowers guard the garden, in our previous example. Suggest depth by including in your picture things of familiar size (people, cars, or an oversized radish or the watermelon of the century placed next to the kid).

Check the direction of light, and walk around to find the right angle. A low angle can make flowers, bushes and that huge pumpkin appear taller. A busy background could mar a photo. It's okay to stage the look with props in order to get the concept you're striving for. Taking photos from a high angle, such as taken from the top of a car or a wall, from a fence or hill, can eliminate gray skies or reveal clouds. According to professional photographers, the failure to get close enough to the subject is one of the most common photography mistakes.

When snapping photos, think about the composition. Centering your subject in the photograph and snapping the shutter isn't composition. It's quick and efficient and dull. Coming up with an eye-stopping photo requires time to arrange your images and practice.

All pictures require a center of interest—a point to which the eye is drawn. But where should you place it? Follow the rule of thirds: Imagine lines dividing your picture into thirds, vertically and horizontally. A good place for the center of interest in any point is where these lines intersect. And check for ground and background clutter, yes, the garbage we've talked about. When photographing people, try focusing on their eyes. Triangular patterns are good for group portraits. Frame your subject with a pleasing background. Don't get stuck in a horizontal mold where everything feels stiff. And when you get bored with these rules, break them.

With candid shots, the photographer doesn't plan but is ready to snap when it happens. Timing is essential; preparation is the key. Try pre-focusing your camera on an area in which you know the action will occur, i.e., the arbor bursting with "Fairy" roses under which a couple will be kissing after the "I do's."

Capture the details of the environment. Include how subjects or animals are involved. For instance, when taking pictures of a therapy garden at a hospital or care facility for the elderly, you might want to pose a child being taught to plant seedlings by one of the senior residents. Be patient. Wait for the subjects to relax.

For groups, regardless of the age, try arranging people around an activity, such as planting trees on Arbor Day or a tot pushing a pretend lawn mower while her parent pushes the real thing. Set the background to tell a story or reveal the activity. Vary the approach. Select an object to be the focal point of the picture and add objects or props to the background.

A book I've found helpful is *Selling Nature Photographs* by Norbert Wu.

Sometimes the fun is getting yourself in the picture. Imagine a photo of you and that award-winning tomato, or one from the year that your zucchini crop threatened to force you out of house and home.

You can do it even without the help of an assistant with these tips.

Use the timer on your camera to take a photo of yourself alone or with a group. Of course, you'll need a camera with a timer mechanism. Familiarize yourself with it before you get ready to go outdoors. Using a tripod, set your camera up and compose the photograph. You can also sit the camera on a wall or sturdy surface if you don't have a tripod.

Taking a group photo? Have someone stand in your place to mark it. If you're alone, mark the garden spot where you're to stand with a leaf or pebble or even an X in the dirt so that when you set the timer you can dash to the correct spot quickly. You might want to put a broom in the spot (if you'll be standing) or a chair, if you're going to be kneeling down as if you're working in the soil. Of course, you'll remove the chair or broom before the shutter clicks.

Now set the timer and move into place and remain in that place until you hear the shutter mechanism click and the picture has been taken. Give yourself about one minute of time to get into place. If you try to do it more quickly, you may end up with a breathless image of yourself. If you have too much time, you may be tempted to move or shift positions just as the shutter clicks.

If you're working with a public therapy garden, documentation can be beneficial to the gardeners, staff members and the media. You need not be a photo genius, but with these tips, you'll be on the way to success.

If you're tempted, don't hesitate. A photo gallery of your garden and the gardens you visit will provide a rich trip down memory lane for you and others.

The fruit of the Spirit is love, joy, peace,
longsuffering, gentleness, goodness,
faith, meekness, temperance.
—Galatians 5:22-23

*You cannot plough a field
by turning it over in your mind.
—Anonymous*

Shovel These Thoughts

There's always work to do in the garden. Regardless of what you attempt, you know in your heart of hearts it could have been better if… It's the "if" that keeps us gardeners gardening because next year it will be better if…

As I finish writing *Shovel It*, I'm looking out at my naked rose garden on an early February afternoon. This book has been with me on a full circle through an entire year, and it's been close to four years since this book's seed was planted in my heart and mind. I thought the book and the concept of *Shovel It* would grow faster, most of my book projects do. The majority of the books I create are written in one season, four months at the most. Silly me. I thought I could force it, much like I do with bulbs in the spring. But in thinking so, I forgot a critical part of gardening. Only Nature knows when things should hibernate, germinate and grow, and when the fruits should be harvested. It's all in God's plan. Nothing happens before the right time. Even for a pushy writer and an impatient gardener like me, the same rules hold true.

Through reading this book, it's my fondest desire and deepest hope that you'll give gardening a chance whenever you're:

Happy

Serious

A bit crazy

A bit too somber

Uneasy

Tired

Excited

Joyful

Unhappy

Unwell

Miffed to beat the band

Out-of-sorts

Perplexed

Blasé

Disjointed

Carefree

Tempted by what the world says is necessary for a perfect life

Relieved

Harassed

Anxious

Silly

Lost

Found

Feeling good

Feeling crummy

Feeling on top of the world

Grief-filled

Hope-filled

Lonely

Pregnant

Empty Nested

Blissful

Disappointed

Regretful

Contented

Overwhelmed

Underwhelmed

Offended

Glad

And in every other mood you feel.

Nature knows what you need and will take care of you if you'll join forces and just *Shovel It*.

Bibliography

Adil, Janeen R. *Accessible Gardening for People with Disabilities*. Bethesda, MD: Woodbine House, 1994.

Barasch, Marc Ian and Caryle Hirshberg. *Remarkable Recovery*. New York: Riverhead Books, 1995.

Bensoussan, A., Talley, N. J., et al. "Chinese Herbs Soothe Irritable Bowel Syndrome," News & Perspectives, *WholeHealthMD*, www.wholehealthmd.com.

Bonica, J.J., ed. *The Management of Cancer Pain*. Philadelphia: Lea & Feiger, 1990.

Cameron, Julia. *The Artist's Way*. New York: Tarcher, 1992.

"Complementary Therapies for Cancer Care," *Mayo Clinic Rochester News*, July 31, 2000.

Cruso, Thalassa. *A Gardening Year*. New York: Lyons & Burford, 1990.

Dennis, Lynn. *Garden for Life*. Saskatchewan, Canada: University Extension Press, University of Saskatchewan, 1994.

Dossey, Larry, M.D. *Reinventing Medicine: Beyond Mind-Body to a New Era of Health*. New York: HarperCollins, 1999.

Duke. *Herbs of the Bible: 2000 Years of Plant Medicine*. Loveland, CO: Interweave Press, 1999

Edell, Dean, MD. "Aromatherapy: Sniffing Out the Science," August 25, 2000, *HealthCentral*, www.healthcentral.com.

Eisenberg, David M., M.D., ed. "Trends in Alternative Medicine Use in the United States, 1990-1997," The *Journal of the American Medical Association*, original contributions November 11, 1998, www.ama-assn.org.

"Exercise Fights Off Depression," *Psychosomatic Medicine*, September 20, 2000, http://onhealth.webmd.com.

Flagler, Joel and Raymond P. Poincelot, eds. *People-Plant Relationships: Setting Research Priorities*. New York: Food Products Press, 1994.

Foley, Tricia. *Having Tea: Recipes & Table Settings*. New York: Clarkson & Potter, 1987.

"Garden Therapy," Anne Jaeger, KOIN-TV, Channel 6000, www.koin.com/athome, Interview with Lauretta Young, Chief of Mental Health at Kaiser Permanente, November 13, 1999.

George, Mike. *Learn to Relax: A Practical Guide to Easing Tension & Conquering Stress*. San Francisco: Chronicle Books, 1999.

Goldman, Bart, M.D. "What Can People Do On their Own to Relieve Chronic Pain," *HealthCentral*, www.healthcentral.com.

Goldman, Connie and Richard Mahler. *Tending the Earth, Mending the Spirit: The Healing Gifts of Gardening*. Center City, MN, Hazelden, 2000

Grad, Bernard R. "Some Biological Effects of Laying-On of the Hands: A Review of Experiments with Animals and Plants," *Journal of The American Society for Psychical Research 59a*, 1965.

Harding, Deborah C. *The Green Guide to Herb Gardening*. St. Paul, MN: Llewellyn Publications, 2000.

Hepper, F. Nigel. *Planting a Bible Garden: A Good Book Practical Guide*. Grand Rapids, MI: Revell Company, 1997.

Jaret P. "The Old Advice: Work out. The New Advice: Walk the Dog and Take the Stairs," *Health*, September 1994.

Krucoff, Carol. "Sculpting Your Muscles and Your Garden," *Los Angeles Times*, August 24, 1998.

Lang, Joseph K. *How to Photograph Landscapes*. Mechanicsburg, PA: Stackpole Books, 1998.

Lemaitre, Rozenn N., Ph.D., MPH, et al. "Leisure-Time Physical Activity and the Risk of Primary Cardiac Arrest," Archives of *Internal Medicine*, James E. Dalen, MD, Editor, www.ama-assn.org, April 12, 1999.

Louden, Jennifer. *The Woman's Comfort Book: A Self-Nurturing Guide for Restoring Balance in Your Life*. New York: Harper Collins, 1992.

"Mary's Gardens", http://www.mgardens.org, Lady Virgin Mary Flower Garden Medieval Catholic Folklore Symbols, 1999.

Activity Therapy, "*Mayo Clinic Health Letter*," August, 1995, page 8.

McCartney, Susan. *Travel Photography*. New York: Allworth, 1992.

Mitchell, Henry. *Henry Mitchell on Gardening*. Boston: Houghton Mifflin, 1998.

O'Hara, MaryAnn, M.D., MST., et al. "A Review of the 12 Commonly Used Medicinal Herbs," Archives of Family Medicine, *Journal of the American Medical Association*, November/December 1998, www.ama-assn.org.

Recer, Paul. "People who exercise brains are less likely to get Alzheimer's," *Seattle Post-Intelligencer*, March 6, 2001.

Relf, Diane. "Horticulture: A Therapeutic Tool," www.hort.vt.edu/human/ht5a.html

Relf, Diane, ed. *The Role of Horticulture in Human Well-Being and Social Development*. Portland, OR: Timber Press, 1992.

Restuccio, Jeffrey P. *Fitness the Dynamic Gardening Way*. Cordova, TN: Balance of Nature Publishing, 1992.

Shaw, Eva, Ph.D. *Writing the Nonfiction Book*. Loveland, CO: Rodgers & Nelsen Publishers, 1999.

Shaw, Eva, Ph.D. *What To Do When A Loved One Dies: A Practical and Compassionate Guide to Dealing with Death on Life's Terms*. Irvine, CA: Dickens Press, 1994.

Terr, Lenore, M.D. *Beyond Love and Work: Why Adults Need to Play*. New York: Scribner, 1999.

Woy, Joann. *Accessible Gardening: Tips and Techniques for Seniors and the Disabled*. Mechanicsburg, PA: Stackpole Books, 1997.

Wu, Norbert. *Selling Nature Photographs*. Mechanicsburg, PA: Stackpole Books, 1997.

Yoemans, Kathleen. *The Able Gardener*. Pownal, VT: Storey Communications, 1992.

Recommended Reading

A Gardener's Bouquet of Quotations, Maria Pulushkin Robbins, editor, Ecco Press, 1993.

Beds I Have Known: Confessions of a Passionate Amateur Gardener, Martha Smith, Moyer Bell Publishing, 1997.

Henry Mitchell on Gardening, Henry Mitchell, Houghton Mifflin, 1998 and all books by Henry Mitchell.

In Search of Lost Roses, Thomas Christopher, Avon, 1989.

Mrs. Greenthumbs Plows Ahead: Five Steps to the Drop-Dead Gorgeous Garden of Your Dreams, Cassandra Danz, Three Rivers, 1998.

People with Dirty Hands: The Passion for Gardening, Robin Chotzinoff, Harcourt Brace, 1996.

Second Nature: A Gardener's Education, Michael Pollan, Delta Books, 1991.

Slug Tossing and Other Adventures of a Reluctant Gardener, Meg Des Camp, Sasquatch Books, 1998.

Sunset Western Landscaping and *Sunset Western Garden Books*, Sunset Books.

About Eva Shaw

Shovel It: Nature's Health Plan is the latest book by Eva Shaw, Ph.D. Writer, speaker, teacher, and gardener, Eva has been publishing for more than twenty years. She has carved out a name in the how-to and self-help categories, including fitness, recovery, gardening and business. She has traveled nationally lecturing on complementary therapies and grief management. Eva is available to speak to groups and can be reached through her website at www.evashaw.com.

With 60 books, more than 1000 magazine articles and columns, and as a full-time writer, Eva teaches writing with Education To Go (a supplier of classes contracted to colleges and universities worldwide via the Internet) and in person with the University of California. She creates curriculum for the Institute of Children's Literature and Long Ridge Writers Group and lectures on writing conferences, colleges, and writing centers throughout the country.

Eva's latest books for writers are *The Successful Writer's Guide to Publishing Magazine Articles* and *Writing the Nonfiction Book*, from the Rodgers & Nelsen Publishers. Other titles include *Insider's Guide to San Diego* (Falcon Publishing), *For the Love of Children* (Health Communications), the award-winning *What to Do When a Loved One Dies* (Dickens Press), *Eve of Destruction* (Contemporary Books), *365 Reflections on Love* and *Marriage and 365 Reflections on Friendship* (Adams Media), and *60-Second Shiatzu* (Henry Holt).

Eva recently completed a coffee table-style book of early California history, The *Sun Never Sets: Influences of the British, Welsh, Irish, Scottish an Canadians on Early California* (Dickens Press).

She has been honored by the Orange County (California) Literacy Guild at the Festival of Women Authors. She is a member of the American Society of Journalists and Authors, Garden Writers Association of America, and the Navy/Marine Relief Society. She's an advocate for issues concerning women and children and an active volunteer with the San Diego Union Rescue Mission, the Florence Crittenton Center, her church and other organizations. Eva is currently "building" a library for residents of the Florence Crittenton Center of Los Angeles.

A resident of Carlsbad, Californian, Eva hikes the world with her husband, Joseph, and plays fetch with Zippy, their ever-energetic Welsh terrier. Eva tends a prize-winning rose garden and cutting gardens, reads, crochets heirloom afghans and makes crafty crafts.